Perfect Por[tions]

How to eat your favour[ite] foods and still lose weight

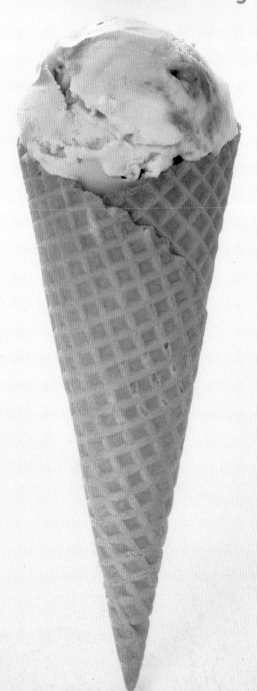

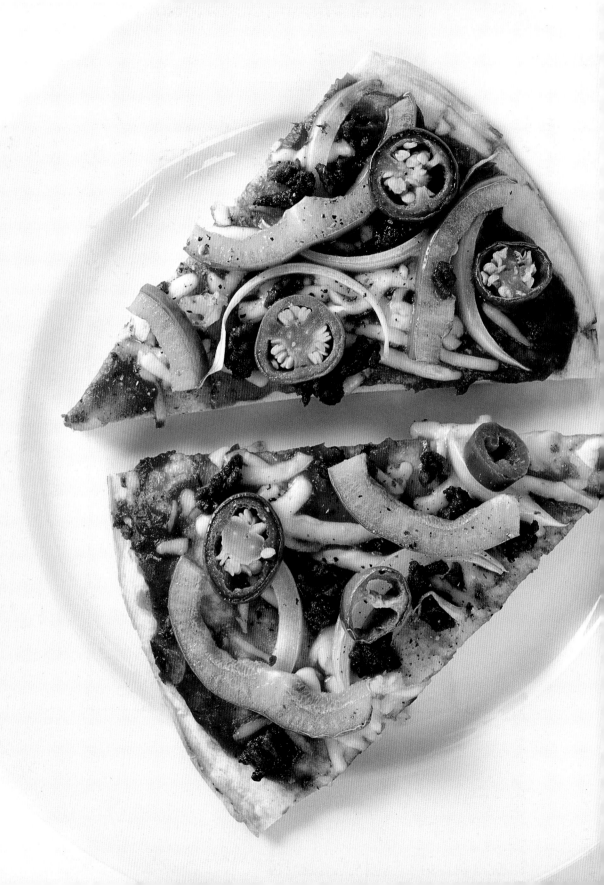

Perfect Portion

How to eat your favourite foods and still lose weight

Linda Gassenheimer

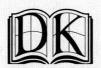

London, New York, Melbourne,
Munich, Delhi

To my husband Harold for his constant
support and love

Project Editor Hilary Mandleberg
Project Designer Ruth Hope
Senior Editor Jennifer Latham
Senior Art Editor Anne Fisher
Managing Editor Penny Warren
Managing Art Editor Marianne Markham
Publishing Operations Manager Gillian Roberts
Creative Publisher Mary-Clare Jerram
Art Director Peter Luff
Publishing Director Corinne Roberts
DTP Designer Sonia Charbonnier
Production Controller Maria Elia

First published in Great Britain in 2007 by
Dorling Kindersley Limited
80 Strand, London WC2R 0RL
Penguin Group (UK)

Copyright © 2007 Dorling Kindersley Limited
Text copyright © 2007 Linda Gassenheimer

2 4 6 8 10 9 7 5 3 1

Note on metric to imperial conversions
The quantities of the foods in this book have been
carefully calculated in grams. Quantities in ounces are
not precise conversions. Use either metric or imperial
measurements, not a mixture of the two. For greatest
accuracy, use the grams measurements.

A CIP catalogue record is available from the
British Library
ISBN 978-1-4053-1739-9

Colour reproduction by Colourscan, Singapore
Printed and bound by Sheck Wah Tong, Hong Kong

Discover more at
www.dk.com

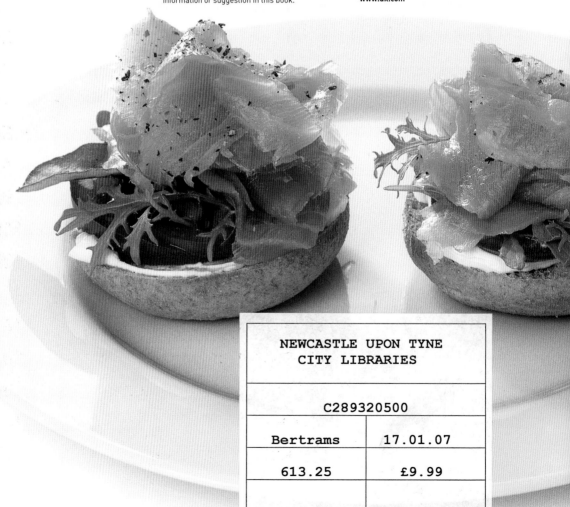

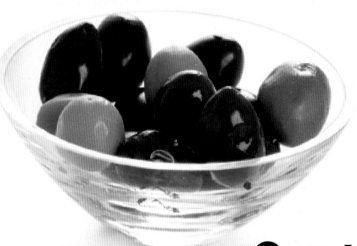

Contents

introduction

Can you have a healthy lifestyle and lose weight without giving up your favourite foods – including chocolate, wine and pasta? Yes, if you follow the guidelines in Perfect Portion. This book shows you the way to a lifetime of good food that doesn't pile on the weight. You don't have to deny yourself. What is a perfect portion? To test your portion IQ, take the quiz on pages 8–11. To fill your IQ gaps, the Portion Guide section shows life-size photos to help you select the right foods in the right portions. How do you fit your choices into your everyday meals? See my Seven-Day Eating Plan for breakfasts, lunches and dinners based on perfect portions. My Eating Out guide shows you how to maintain your portion plan for a wide variety of ethnic foods. Enjoy this book and great food that's good for you, too.

Portion quiz

How many times do you choose a plate of fried chicken for dinner, a filled baked potato as a side dish or a 120g (4¼oz) bowl of cereal for breakfast? Do you think you're eating a healthy, nutritious meal? And what about those snacks? Do you truly know how many calories you're having when you sit in front of the TV and dip into that bag of crisps? To see if you really suffer from portion distortion, take a moment to test yourself with this fun-to-do quiz. Be prepared for some surprises!

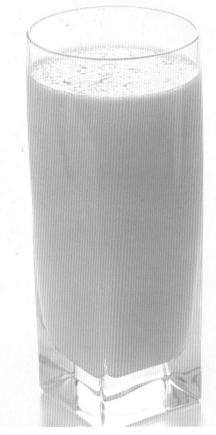

1 A 355ml (12fl oz) glass of orange juice like this is good for you isn't it?

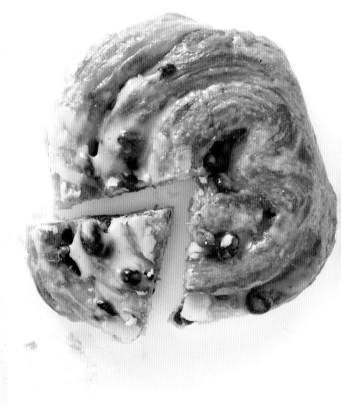

2 How does that Danish pastry you picked up for breakfast measure up?

3 Which meal would you prefer: a large helping of fried chicken or a steak dinner?

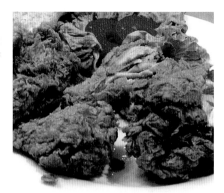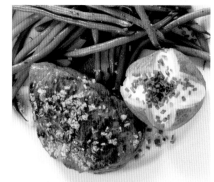

4 Which of these two bagels do you think is the healthy one? The one with the seeds on top, or the one with the smoked salmon?

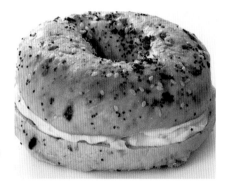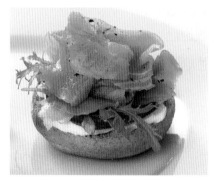

5 You crave a baked potato but how much should you be eating, and what should you choose to top it?

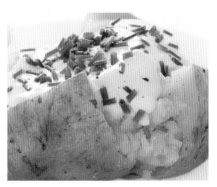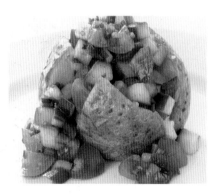

6 Which of these chips will give you around half of your daily calories? The 198g (7oz) serving or the 85g (3oz) one?

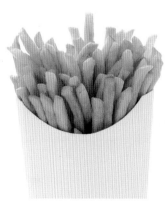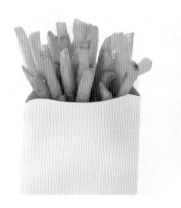

7 How many calories do you think are in this sandwich? Might it be 200, 400, 600 or 800?

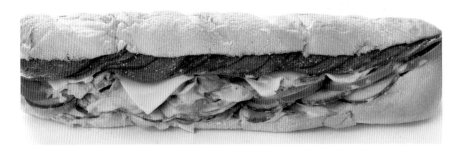

8 Surely a person can have that healthy granola on the left for their cereal? Why bother with the granola, yogurt and almonds?

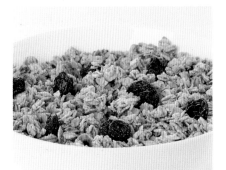
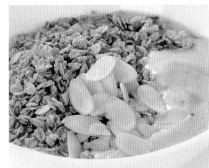

9 Do you regularly order four fat slices of a big pizza with all the toppings you can? Have you any idea how many calories they contain?

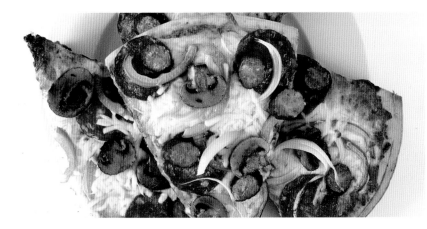

10 What's your best bet for a mid-afternoon or evening snack: popcorn, crisps or peanuts?

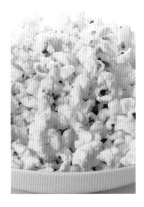
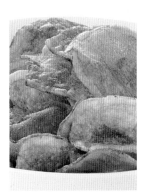
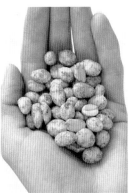

Answers

1 Yes, it is as it will give you some of your daily fruit requirement, but you'll also be getting 168 sugar-packed calories and almost no fibre. It would be better to drink half that amount of juice – and better still to eat the fruit itself.

2 You thought that 135g (4¾oz) Danish pastry was harmless but it has 520 calories with 28g of fat and it's packed with sugar. Not a good start to the day.

3 Have you chosen the fried chicken? Deep-fried foods add calories and fat. A 454g (16oz) serving (without bones) of fried chicken can add up to about 1200 calories. Instead, enjoy the balanced steak dinner and have 88g (3oz) of raspberry sorbet as dessert. That will give you a total of about 570 calories.

4 The 11cm (4½in) bagel with 57g (2oz) of cream cheese equals 560 calories. The 5cm (2in) bagel with cream cheese, smoked salmon, lettuce and tomato has only 320 calories. Add 30g (1oz) bran cereal with 118ml (4fl oz) skimmed milk for 423 calories for a breakfast with good nutritional value.

5 Potatoes are good for us but that large baked potato with butter and soured cream weighs in at 578 calories. The smaller one with salsa is about 136 calories and has less fat. It also gives you extra healthy vegetables.

6 This typical large 198g (7oz) serving of chips weighs in at a whopping 660 calories or almost half your daily calorie allowance. The small portion of 85g (3oz) is about 210 calories.

7 This 30cm (12in) sandwich will set you back by more than 800 calories. That's more than half what most of us should be eating in a whole day.

8 Just 204g (7¼oz) of granola add up to about 800 calories. A smaller portion of low-fat granola topped with fat-free, low-sugar, flavoured yogurt, and with a sprinkling of almonds on top, comes in at only 415 calories and is much healthier for you, too.

9 Eat all this pizza with a bottle of beer and you'll be having at least 2000 shocking calories. That's part of tomorrow's calorie allowance, too!

10 A large tub of popcorn has over 600 calories plus a lot of salt. A 113g (4oz) bag of crisps is about 600 calories. The best choice is peanuts. They have monounsaturated fat and protein, while dry-roasted peanuts have only 170 calories per 28g (1oz). That's about 40 peanuts.

The science behind portion control

I've been working with a number of endocrinologists, cardiologists and registered dieticians for over ten years on the growing, world-wide problem of obesity. Many factors have been quietly undermining people's struggle to keep their weight down.

The first is that we are not selecting the right foods to eat and the second is that the portions of foods we are eating have ballooned. Restaurants serve extra-large amounts of food, yet we still clean our plates, just as we were told to do when we were children. Fast-food portions have also grown – up two to five times over twenty years.

Research findings

A growing body of research shows that most people are blissfully unaware of how much food is being put in front of them. At Pennsylvania State University, researchers found that people tended to eat whatever was on their plate or in a serving package. Using macaroni cheese and 30cm (12in) sandwiches as 'test' foods, the researchers found that adults ate at least 30 per cent more calories when larger portions of these foods were put in front of them – even though they generally were just as satisfied by the smaller portions.

 Package size makes a difference, too. The same researchers found that women given a 454g (1lb) box of spaghetti to make a dinner for two

> Most people are unaware of how much food is being put in front of them

The difference between a portion and a serving

This book is about portion size – the amount of each type of food that you choose to eat to make up a meal or snack, whether you are at home or in a restaurant. A serving, however, is a standard amount that is used, for example, for calculating recipe serving quantities, for diet plans and for cookery books. Serving sizes are given on the Nutrition Facts labels on packaged foods. Beware. A serving size is not necessarily the same as the amount in the package. You need to read the labels carefully.

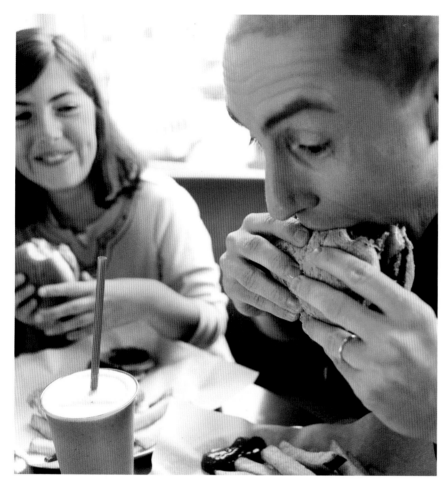

The increase of size in fast-food portions is one of the reasons we are fatter than ever before. Not only is the food often chock-full of calories and saturated fat, but we also eat it too frequently. Ask yourself how many times a week you stop at a fast-food restaurant for a quick meal for yourself or your family – then you might see why you struggle to keep your weight down.

removed an average of 234 strands. But if they were given a 900g (2lb) box and told to make the same dinner, they removed an average of 302 strands – 29 per cent more.

Other studies that used crisps and sweets have shown drastic increases in snacking when the subject was given a larger amount of food to dip into.

So, how can you picture what you should eat and what portions you should be eating? In the pages of Perfect Portion you'll find the answers at a glance. The book is organized to show you the good (choices to savour), the bad (choices to watch) and the ugly (choices to avoid). For example, in the meat, fish and dairy sections, I show you how to select foods with lean protein and how to avoid large amounts of saturated fat. In the grains and vegetables and fruit sections, I show you how to select foods that are high in complex carbohydrates. Throughout the book I show you how to add monounsaturated fat to your diet.

Be plate wise...

At the same time as portions and package sizes have grown, the size of the plates and bowls we eat from has grown too. You used to have your dinner on a 25cm (10in) plate, but often it's a 30cm (12in) plate or larger these days. You still fill your cereal bowl to the top, but did you notice the size of the bowl that came with the set of tableware you bought the other day?

That bowl is probably 20cm (8in) across, while the old one was only 15cm (6in). Even dishwashers are now designed to hold larger plates and bowls.

So why does any of this matter? Because we can now get even more food on our plates and in our bowls. And, as the research has shown, once we do that, we eat more without realizing it. One friend mentioned to me that she gained 2.27kg (5lb) after buying a dinner service with restaurant-size dinner plates. It sounds crazy but it's true.

With a 25cm (10in) plate, overweight will soon be a thing of the past

Corral your breakfast calories into a 15cm (6in) bowl and you'll control your waistline

25cm (10in) plate

15cm (6in) bowl

...and drinks savvy

The bad news doesn't stop at plates and bowls. Our cups and glasses have ballooned in size, too, which means we're drinking more than we once did – and we're getting used to it as well, which means we no longer notice.

Take drinking glasses for example. If you have those big, 355ml (12fl oz) glasses, save them for water. A 237ml (8fl oz) glass is large enough for most drinks. A 177ml (6fl oz) glass is best for juice. And stick to a 237ml (8fl oz) cup or mug for your tea or coffee with milk. That way you won't be consuming lots of extra calories.

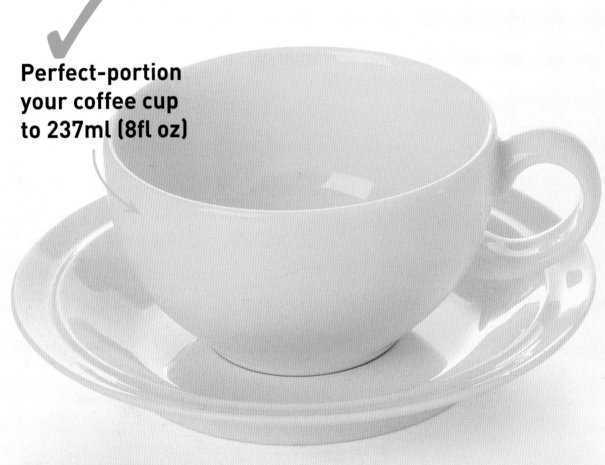

**Perfect-portion
your coffee cup
to 237ml (8fl oz)**

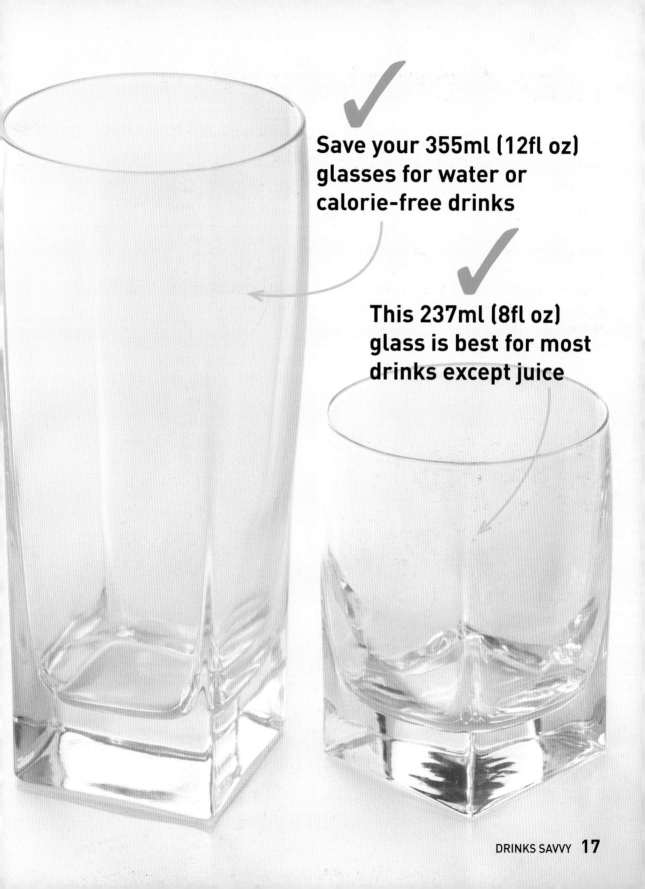

✓ Save your 355ml (12fl oz) glasses for water or calorie-free drinks

✓ This 237ml (8fl oz) glass is best for most drinks except juice

The benefits of not being overweight

Whatever our age, we all want to enjoy life to the full.
The best way to achieve that goal is to stay healthy, so keep
your weight down by selecting the right foods and eating them
in the right portions – this book will show you how – and by
exercising regularly. And if you're seeking the fountain of
youth, watching your weight can help stop the clock, too.

There's no doubt that being the correct weight for your sex and age
improves your health. Likely benefits are lowering your cholesterol as well
as your blood-sugar and blood-pressure levels. This, in turn, can decrease
your chances of suffering from serious disabling diseases such as stroke,
diabetes, heart disease, arthritis and cancer. Losing only 10 per cent of
your body weight has been shown to lower blood pressure and blood-
sugar levels and to mitigate the symptoms of pre-diabetes.

Measuring your BMI

A high percentage of body fat is an indicator of overweight. The best way to measure your body-
fat percentage is to use the Body Mass Index (BMI). Below is the formula for calculating your BMI
if your weight is in kilograms. If your weight is in pounds, you need to multiply the result by 703.

$$BMI = \frac{\text{weight in kilograms}}{\text{height in metres squared}}$$

For example, to find the BMI of a 68kg (150lb) person who is 1.65m (5'5") tall:

$$BMI = \frac{68}{(1.65 \times 1.65)} = 24.9 \text{ BMI}$$

A BMI of between 19 and 24.9 is considered normal.
A BMI of 25 or over is considered overweight.

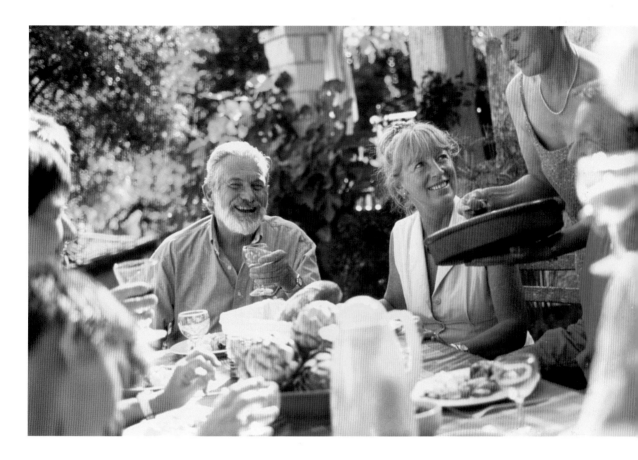

Control your portion sizes, eat a healthy diet and exercise regularly. That way you can enjoy life to the full and help keep serious disabling diseases at bay.

Another significant factor to consider is the diminished quality of life that inevitably comes from being overweight. You may have breathing problems and sleep apnoea. Indulgent eating and lack of exercise will decrease your energy. You feel tired, your skin looks dull and your muscles sag. Tasks tend to become a chore instead of a pleasure. Just thirty minutes' exercise a day can help.

In addition to improving your health, there's a clear financial reason for losing weight: the rising cost of prescriptions and health insurance are a strong incentive to stay well.

Caution

Perfect Portion is intended for everyone who leads a normal lifestyle. Athletes, very active people and those with special medical needs and diets may find that their requirements are different. If you fall into one of these categories or have any other concerns, check with your GP before you modify your eating habits. In fact, it is best for everyone to check with their GP before modifying their eating habits.

Balanced eating

Are you struggling with calorie confusion? We know we should eat between 1400 and 2000 calories a day depending on our size and physical activity. But does this mean we can have muffins for breakfast, biscuits for lunch and cake for supper – all adding up to 1400 calories? The answer is obviously 'no'.

Calories are important, but what is more important is the type of calories. Where should these calories come from? The jury is no longer out. Studies have given us a wealth of information regarding the types of foods we need to eat. One of these, the Nurses' Health Study compiled by the Harvard School of Public Health in the United States, is a key source. In addition, the United States government has compiled a useful food pyramid that gives portion information for a wide variety of different foods.

What to aim for

All these sources agree. We should concentrate on eating lean protein from meat, poultry, fish or shellfish. This should make up a quarter of our plate. Another quarter should be whole grains such as wholemeal bread, whole-wheat pasta and brown rice, which are excellent sources of slowly digested, fibre-filled complex carbohydrates.

Vegetables and fruit are good sources of proteins and carbohydrates but are often neglected. Aim to fill the other half of your plate with vegetables and have at least 220–340g (7³⁄₄–12oz) of fruit a day. Vegetables and fruit will add essential vitamins, minerals and fibre to your diet.

And where do fats and oils come in? Use monounsaturated oils (olive oil and rapeseed oil) and keep your saturated fats down to 14–20g daily, depending on your calorie intake. Trans fats (or trans fatty acids) – created by the partial hydrogenation of vegetable oils and found in many processed foods – should be avoided.

My Seven-Day Eating Plan (*see pages 160–180*) shows you how to eat balanced meals every day of the week, without breaking the portion plan bank. It contains the right proportions of lean protein, complex carbs and monounsaturated fat. Follow the plan and once you're familiar with 'eyeballing' correct-sized portions – which is the unique feature of Perfect Portion – you can start to make clever substitutions to suit your own tastes.

Perfect Portion helps you eat a balanced diet

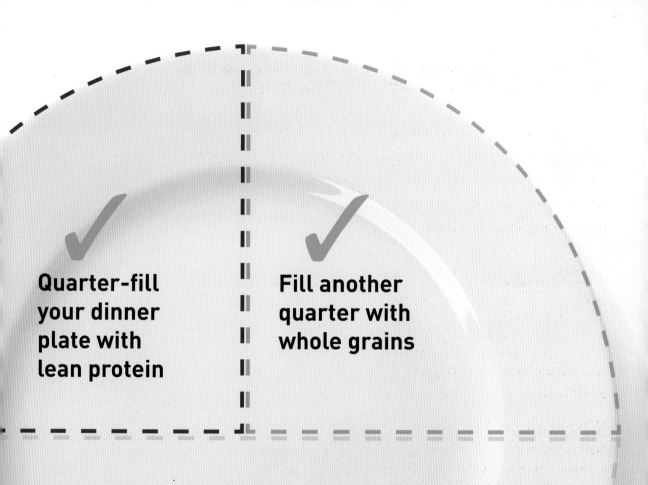

Quarter-fill your dinner plate with lean protein

Fill another quarter with whole grains

Half a plate of vegetables adds nutrients and fibre to your diet

Having a bad day? X

If you laid out your day's breakfast, lunch, dinner, drinks and snacks on a table, might they look like this? This food is actually enough for five people.

Pour yourself 82g (3oz) of this cereal and have this 570ml (20fl oz) speciality coffee with whipped cream for 1000 calories.

A typical buffet lunch with buttered white bread and a 710ml (24fl oz) regular cola is a real sugar-and-saturated-fat fest.

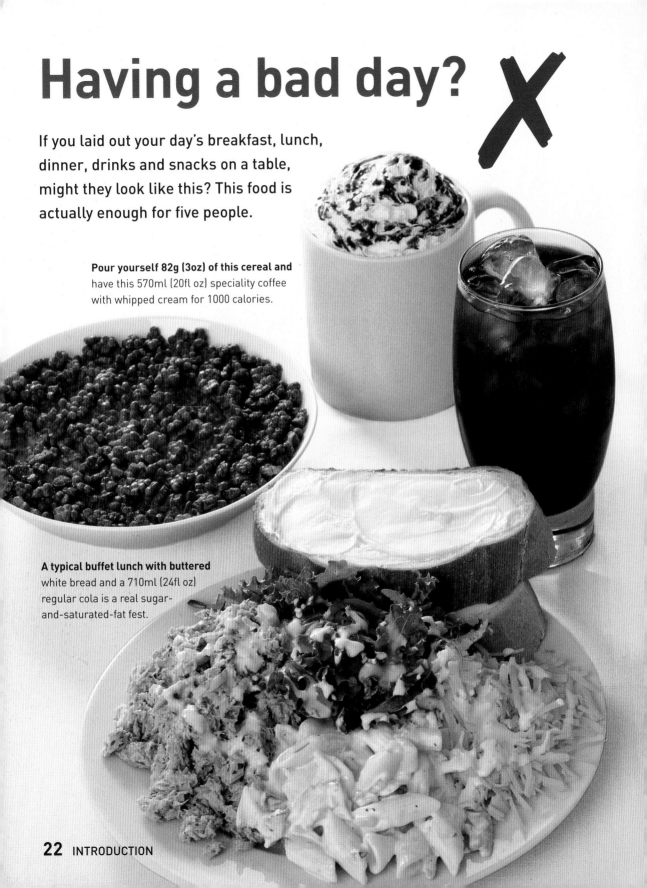

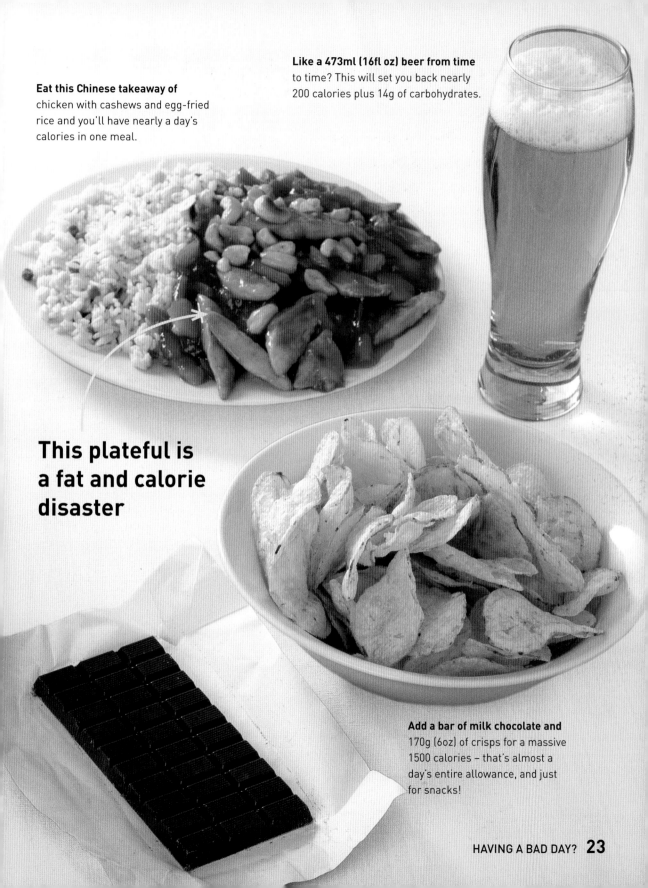

Eat this Chinese takeaway of chicken with cashews and egg-fried rice and you'll have nearly a day's calories in one meal.

Like a 473ml (16fl oz) beer from time to time? This will set you back nearly 200 calories plus 14g of carbohydrates.

This plateful is a fat and calorie disaster

Add a bar of milk chocolate and 170g (6oz) of crisps for a massive 1500 calories – that's almost a day's entire allowance, and just for snacks!

Have a nice day

Want to eat a more healthy diet and keep your portions under control? Then this is what your day's food should look like. Eyeball the portions in this book. The pictures are not only worth a thousand words, they will save you thousands of calories.

Lunch is a tasty Greek salad (*recipe, page 170*) with a 355ml (12fl oz) diet drink.

Have this low-fat granola cereal breakfast (*recipe, page 170*) with a 237ml (8fl oz) coffee with skimmed milk for 430 calories.

Eyeball these pictures to save over

4000

calories a day

Fancy a glass of wine with dinner? This 148ml (5fl oz) glass of red wine comes in at only 106 calories.

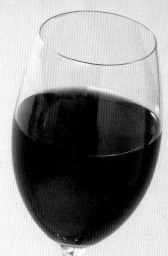

Delicious Chicken Provençal with spinach lentils (*recipes, page 171*) are a healthy dinner choice.

You can still enjoy your snacks – just stick to 28g (1oz) portions.

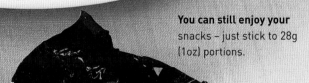

Tips for eating less

You know you should eat smaller portions and be a healthy weight. But it can be difficult. We buy many different foods and eat in many different places, each with its own temptations. Here are some tips to help you stick to your perfect portions whatever the situation.

Eat high quality, low quantity Real food with great flavour is more satisfying than diet or convenience foods that are filled with chemicals. You'll feel fuller and won't reach for the packet of biscuits ten minutes after you've eaten.

Make time to eat It takes twenty minutes for your stomach to signal to your brain that you're full. Put your fork down between bites. This will give you time to really taste and enjoy your food.

Turn off the TV or computer Watching the TV or working on the computer while you're eating is a sure-fire way of expanding your waistline. Your plate might be clean before you realize you've eaten a meal.

Have a snack mid-morning and mid-afternoon The ideal meal plan is to have three balanced meals and two snacks a day. About 28g (1oz) of

The symbols used in this book

We have chosen symbols showing different parts of the hand to indicate how much of each food makes the perfect portion. These are based on roughly how that food will appear on the plate in front of you and they will help you to 'eyeball' the correct portions. Obviously we all have different size hands. The best way for you to create your own personal symbols is to compare your hand to the life-size photos in this book. Our guidelines will help you get started.

 palm

 cupped hand

 fist

 thumb

 hand

 cupped hands

 finger

 thumb tip

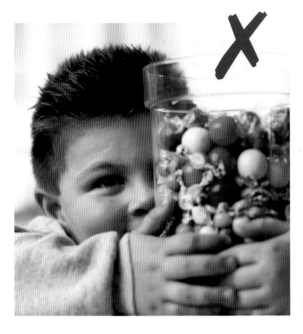

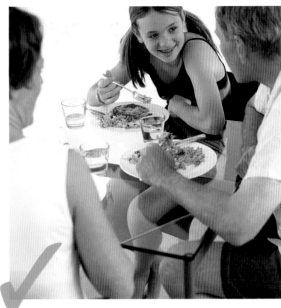

Start young and give your children good habits. Make it a rule that they don't eat straight from the container. Instead, measure out their portion. And gather around the table for family mealtimes. Everyone will enjoy their meal more and will feel satisfied for longer.

either almonds, pecans or walnuts, 123g (4½oz) fat-free yogurt, or a helping of raw vegetables such as celery, carrots, broccoli or cauliflower florets all make great snacks.

Eat as a family Try to sit down to dinner as a family. The focus on conversation and the day's events helps you relax and savour your dinner.

Portion out your snack foods For example, divide a 283g (10oz) packet of nuts into ten small plastic bags. Make sure you eat only one bag at a sitting, and put the rest away where you can't see them.

Don't eat out of the bag or container Take the food out of the bag or container and put it in a bowl. That way you can see exactly how much you're eating.

Eat foods that are filling Eating more vegetables with your meal will help fill you up on good-for-you food and will stop you reaching for some junk food half an hour later.

Watch the extras at parties Watch the nibbles and alcohol as they add unnecessary calories. Start with a diet drink or sparkling water, as alcohol increases your appetite. Space out the nibbles that get passed round and have two to three only. Don't stand by the buffet table and talk to a friend. Before you know it, you'll have downed 500 calories or more (*see also Portion distortion: buffet food, pages 158–159*).

At the supermarket Don't shop on an empty stomach. Make a list of exactly what you need and stick to it. Buy enough vegetables to last for a week. Avoid the bargain – buying large-size packages isn't a bargain if they cost you a new pair of jeans.

The importance of exercise

Exercise counts. Being active is an important element to add to your Perfect Portion plan as it helps to burn the calories in your food and keeps that excess weight at bay. The more vigorous your exercise, the more calories you burn. Walking on a treadmill at 4 miles per hour burns 6.6 calories a minute. Swimming breast stroke at a reasonably energetic pace uses 9 calories a minute. Shopping only uses around 4 calories a minute. Strolling doesn't count at all.

You don't need more than 30 minutes a day to add some serious physical activity to your life without even noticing it. You can raise your heart rate by walking, gardening, climbing stairs, or even by dancing the night away. Any of these everyday activities can help you achieve your 30-minutes-a-day exercise goal.

In addition to using calories, physical activity helps maintain your bones, muscles and joints in good condition. It also lowers your risk of coronary heart disease, type 2 diabetes and colon cancer. And it helps to relieve stress and gives you a feeling of wellbeing.

Which exercise to choose

The harder you exercise, the more you'll increase your heart rate and the faster you'll burn those calories. The following will give you an idea of what constitutes moderate and vigorous types of exercise. Before you start any exercise regime, always check with your health professional that you are fit enough to exercise.

Moderate exercise
- Walking briskly at about 3½ miles per hour.
  This can be broken up into two 15-minute sessions if you wish.
- Gardening
- Weight training
- Going for a hike

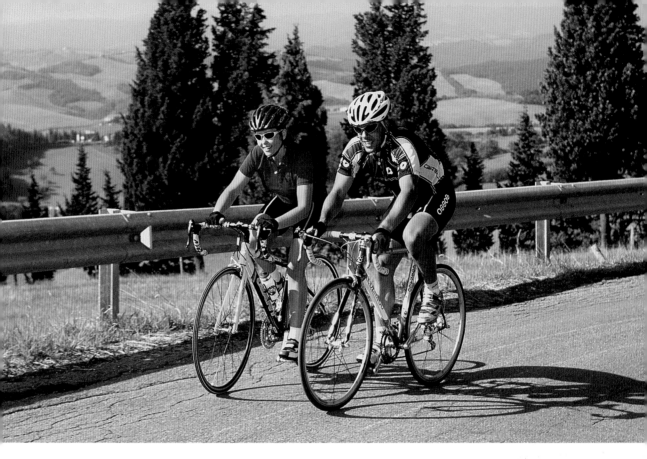

Cycling is a great form of exercise. Not only does it burn calories, but it also gets you out in the open air. Cycling for half an hour at around 5 miles per hour burns an average of 130 calories. If you increase your speed to 9 miles per hour, you'll burn nearly 200 calories.

Vigorous exercise

- Running or jogging at 5 miles per hour
- Walking fast at $4\frac{1}{2}$ miles per hour
- Tennis
- Football
- Swimming (freestyle laps)
- Aerobics

Finding time to exercise

Don't know how you're ever going to fit that all-important exercise into your busy schedule? These tips will help you do it:

- Whenever possible, use the stairs instead of the lift.
- Park your car at the end of the car park instead of in the nearest spot and walk to where you're going as if you were caught in the rain.
- Walk to the golf course carrying your own clubs.
- Ride an exercise bike indoors or cycle to work.
- Vary the times and types of your exercise. Take the dog for a 10-minute walk; take a walk at lunch time for 10 minutes; do some weight training while you're watching TV.

portion guides

- meat and poultry

- fish and shellfish

- dairy

- vegetables and fruit

- grains

- sweet treats

- drinks and snacks

- eating out

meat and poultry

Enjoy your steak, pork or lamb. Lean cuts of these, along with chicken, turkey and certain deli meats, are excellent sources of protein. You should have some protein with each meal. It makes you feel satisfied and will help stop those between-meal cravings. Follow the suggestions here and you won't have to guess what types of meat to buy, the healthiest ways to cook them or the amount to eat without breaking your calorie bank. If you are vegetarian or simply like to have a meat-free day from time to time, see the vegetarian options in this section and the sections on vegetables and grains, which provide dietary protein, too. To discover how to incorporate the foods from this section in your perfect portion plan, see my Seven-Day Eating Plan on pages 160–180.

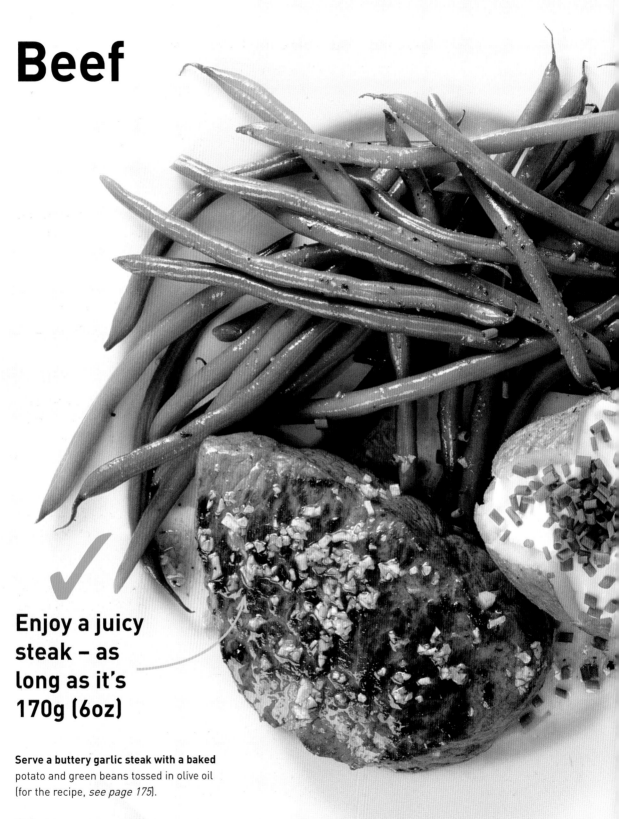

Beef

Enjoy a juicy steak – as long as it's 170g (6oz)

Serve a buttery garlic steak with a baked potato and green beans tossed in olive oil (for the recipe, *see page 175*).

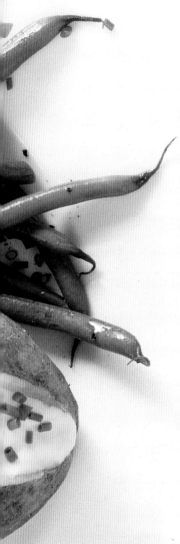

Beef, especially steak, is a favourite for special occasions or for a quick, delicious weekday meal. Enjoy your beef, but beware of your portion size, especially when eating out. A restaurant serving of a 284g (10oz) rib-eye steak can be as much as 780 calories, with 25.5g of saturated fat.

How much can I eat?
Plan on a 170g (6oz) portion of uncooked meat (142g/5oz cooked) after all the visible fat has been removed. A portion like this averages 250 calories with 35 per cent fat.

Cuts to savour
Not all beef is the same. The healthiest cuts are these: Chuck steak • Fillet steak • Flank steak • Porterhouse • Sirloin steak • T-bone • Topside steak

Cuts to watch
A 170g (6oz) uncooked portion (142g/5oz cooked) of these slightly fattier cuts has about 275 calories with 46 per cent fat: Brisket • Rib-eye steak • Rump steak • Skirt • Avoid prime rib joints – a 170g (6oz) portion has about 654 calories with 82 per cent fat

Cooking for health
Always remove all visible fat before cooking to minimize your fat intake. The healthiest ways to cook your beef are to roast, sauté, grill or barbecue it.

Minced beef – check the labels
Labelling for minced beef can be misleading so check carefully to see the fat content. Look for lean minced beef with 20 per cent fat and 63 calories per 28g (1oz) and extra-lean minced beef with 5 per cent fat and only 33 calories per 28g (1oz).

Nutritional analysis
per 170g (6oz) beef steak portion as pictured

234 calories, with 33 per cent from fat; **8.5g** fat, of which **3.0g** saturated fat; **36.1g** protein; **102mg** cholesterol; **96mg** sodium; **0g** fibre
(*see page 178 for nutritional analysis of whole dinner*)

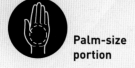

Palm-size portion

Want to eat

800

**calories in one go?
Here's how!**

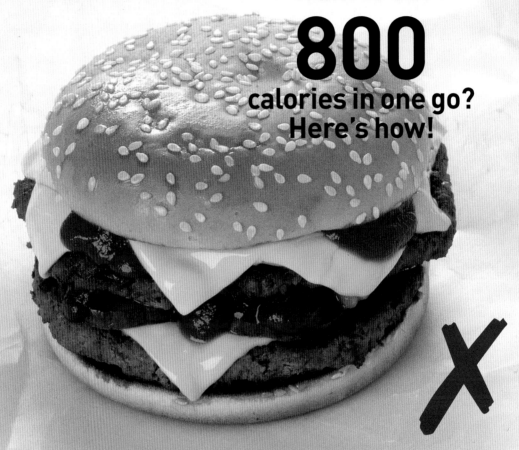

X

oversize portion

Over the years hamburgers have grown from an 85g (3oz) burger with a roll to match weighing in at about 300 calories, to one that is 170–227g (6–8oz), with a large roll. That 170g (6oz) burger weighs in at almost 600 calories. Turn it into a 227g (8oz) cheeseburger with mayonnaise, pickle, ketchup, onion, tomato and lettuce – like the cheeseburger pictured here – and you'll be eating a hefty 800 calories.

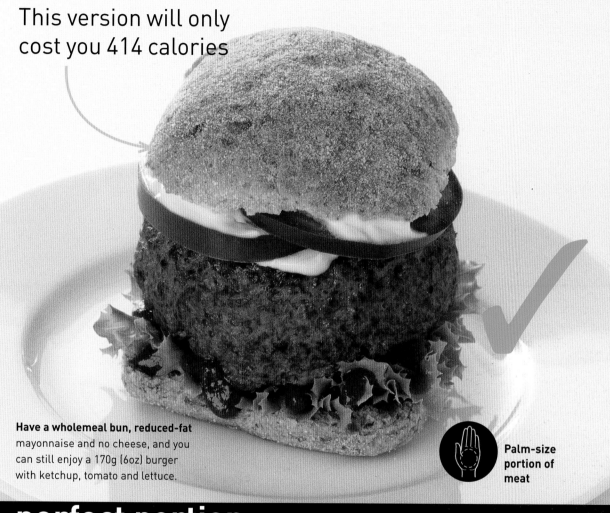

This version will only
cost you 414 calories

Have a wholemeal bun, reduced-fat mayonnaise and no cheese, and you can still enjoy a 170g (6oz) burger with ketchup, tomato and lettuce.

Palm-size portion of meat

perfect portion

Skip the cheese completely and limit yourself to a hamburger made from 170g (6oz) of extra-lean meat (142g/5oz cooked) for dinner. Put it in a 28g (1oz) wholemeal roll and add 1 tbsp ketchup, 1 tbsp reduced-fat mayonnaise, 2 slices of tomato and a large leaf of lettuce, as shown here. You'll only be getting 414 calories. What's more, eating your burger in this wholemeal roll will add some essential whole grains to your diet.

Nutritional analysis
per 170g (6oz) hamburger as pictured

414 calories; **34** per cent fat, **15.5g** fat, of which, **4.9g** saturated fat; **41.6g** protein; **113mg** cholesterol; **617mg** sodium; **3.7g** fibre

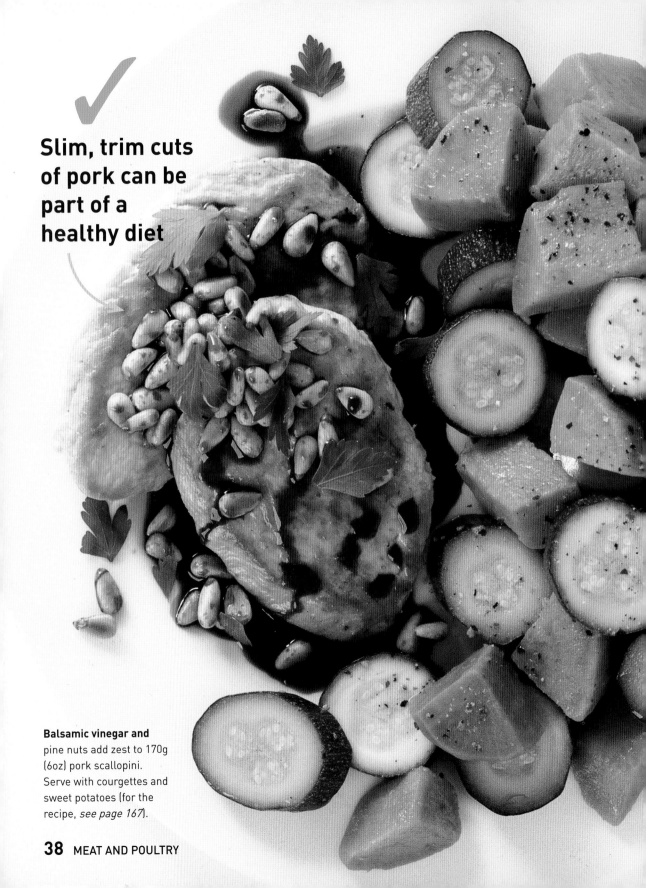

Slim, trim cuts of pork can be part of a healthy diet

Balsamic vinegar and pine nuts add zest to 170g (6oz) pork scallopini. Serve with courgettes and sweet potatoes (for the recipe, *see page 167*).

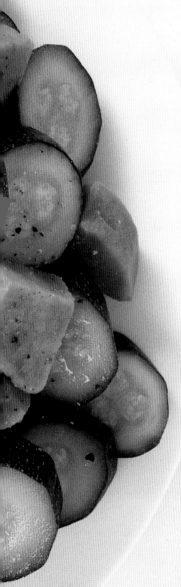

Pork

Pork, now advertised as the other white meat, is a great protein choice, but take care to choose the right cut and the correct portion size. Eat a slab of pork spareribs consisting of about 340g (12oz) of meat and you're having 1260 calories, with 72 per cent from fat.

How much can I eat?
Plan on a 170g (6oz) portion of uncooked meat (142g/5oz cooked), which is about 210 calories and 28 per cent fat.

Choices to savour
Your best pork choices are: Boneless loin chops • Tenderloin • Cured lean ham

Choices to watch
A 170g (6oz) uncooked portion (142g/5oz cooked) of the following slightly fattier cuts has about 252 calories and 41 per cent fat: Boneless loin roast • Back bacon • Pork shoulder

Choices to avoid
A 170g (6oz) portion of pork rinds has from 420 to 930 calories (depending on the variety) and about 70 per cent fat. You should also avoid: Regular (not lean) smoked or cured ham • Bacon • Pork sausage

Healthy ways to enjoy
Remove all visible fat before cooking and skim the fat from the pan juices. Note: the leaner cuts of pork can become dry and tough if overcooked.

Nutritional analysis
per 170g (6oz) pork portion as pictured

204 calories, with 26 per cent from fat; **5.8g** fat, of which, **2g** saturated fat; **35.7g** protein; **108mg** cholesterol; **84mg** sodium; **0g** fibre
(see page 177 for nutritional analysis of whole plate)

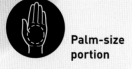

Palm-size portion

Lamb

Lamb is an ingredient in many different cuisines. The aroma of kebabs or butterflied leg of lamb cooking on the grill or barbecue is hard to resist. Leg of lamb roasted in the oven is another delicious way to eat this meat. You can enjoy your lamb, but it's a fatty meat choice, so watch the cuts and make sure to trim off all the visible fat.

How much can I eat?

Plan on having a 170g (6oz) portion of lean, uncooked meat (142g/5oz cooked), which is about 340g (12oz) with the bone and the fat. This averages 220 calories with 35 per cent from fat.

Choices to savour

The healthiest lamb choices are these: Leg—choose from chump end, shank end or 10mm (½in)-thick round steaks cut right through the leg, leaving a small bone in the centre • Shoulder • Kebabs, cut from the leg or shoulder • Loin chops

Choices to avoid

A 170g (6oz) portion of lamb rib chops has 290 calories with 49 per cent from fat.

Healthy ways to enjoy

As with other meats, always cut off all the visible fat. Lean lamb is healthiest for you when it's grilled, barbecued or roasted. You know it's cooked when a meat thermometer reaches 63°C (145°F) for medium-rare or 71°C (160°F) for medium.

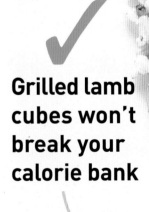

Grilled lamb cubes won't break your calorie bank

Nutritional analysis
per 170g (6oz) lamb portion as pictured

228 calories, with 36 per cent from fat; **9g** fat, of which, **3.2g** saturated fat; **34.4g** protein; **108mg** cholesterol; **108mg** sodium; **0g** fibre
(*see page 176 for nutritional analysis of whole plate*)

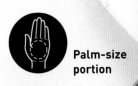

Palm-size portion

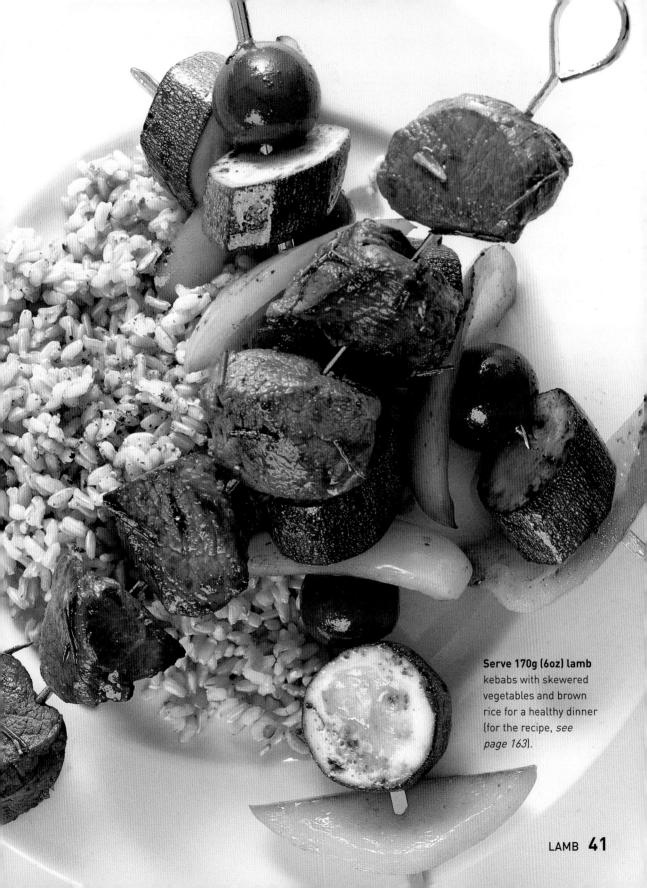

Serve 170g (6oz) lamb kebabs with skewered vegetables and brown rice for a healthy dinner (for the recipe, *see page 163*).

Poultry

'You can never write too many chicken recipes,' one of my editors once told me. Chicken is the most popular meat and turkey is another great choice, since it's the leanest meat you can buy. Watch duck, however. A 227g (8oz) serving of roast duck has 920 calories, with 87 per cent from fat.

How much can I eat?
For chicken and turkey, plan on 170g (6oz) of uncooked boneless white meat (142g/5oz cooked), which has about 186 calories with 10 per cent fat for chicken, 4 per cent fat for turkey. Or plan on 170g (6oz) of uncooked boneless dark meat (142g/5oz cooked), which has 210 calories with 30 per cent from fat.

Choices to savour
Your best poultry choices are: Boneless, skinless chicken breast and thighs • Boneless, skinless turkey breast and thighs

Choices to watch
Enjoy 170g (6oz) of uncooked duck with skin and visible fat removed

Choices to avoid
You should avoid eating: Duck, chicken, and turkey with skin and fat • Chicken wings • Deep-fried chicken

Healthy ways to enjoy
Remove skin and visible fat before serving poultry. Sear boneless, skinless chicken or turkey breast 2 minutes per side, then lower the heat and cook until 77°C (170°F) on the meat thermometer.

Nutritional analysis
per 170g (6oz) chicken portion as pictured

186 calories, with 10 per cent from fat; **2.1g** fat, of which, **0.6g** saturated fat; **39.2g** protein; **96mg** cholesterol; **108mg** sodium; **0g** fibre
(*see page 178 for nutritional analysis of whole plate*)

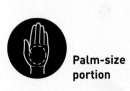

Palm-size portion

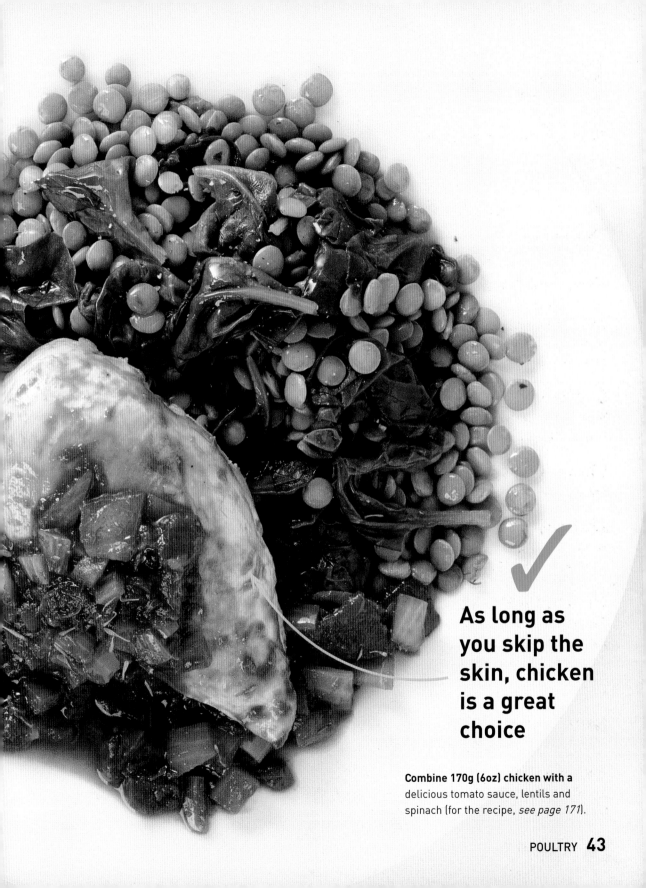

As long as you skip the skin, chicken is a great choice

Combine 170g (6oz) chicken with a delicious tomato sauce, lentils and spinach (for the recipe, *see page 171*).

Deli meats

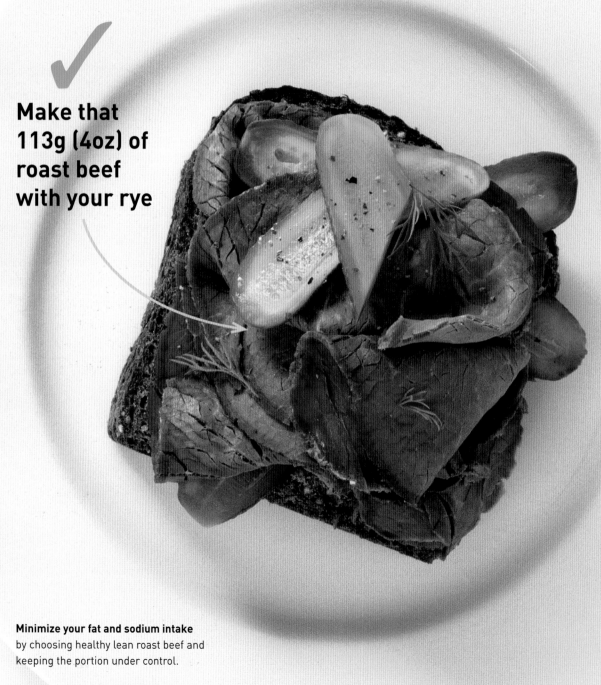

✓

Make that 113g (4oz) of roast beef with your rye

Minimize your fat and sodium intake
by choosing healthy lean roast beef and
keeping the portion under control.

Pick up a ham and Swiss on rye from the deli for lunch and before you eat the pickle that comes with it, you could be having over 1400 calories and 90g of fat, as well as over 5g of sodium. Ordering at a restaurant can be just as damaging. Many restaurants want to give you your money's worth so they overfill their sandwiches with meat and mayonnaise.

How much can I eat?

You should be eating 113g (4oz) of meat or about four slices, but most sandwiches have double that. And keep in mind that processed meats can be filled with sodium. If you're buying at the sandwich bar, ask to see the nutritional analysis of the meat they are using. If it's not available, you can find the information for many brands online. If you are buying pre-packaged deli meat, watch the serving size on the packet. Some labels use a one-slice serving size or about 28g (1oz), while others use 57–85g (2–3oz).

Choices to savour

Some processed meats have an unhealthy 28–36g fat per 113g (4oz) portion. Look for these healthy choices: Skinless, 'lower-sodium' turkey breast averages 30 calories, 0.2g fat and 170mg sodium per 28g (1oz) • Skinless oven-roasted chicken breast averages 30 calories, 0.5 fat and 175mg sodium per 28g (1oz) • Lean roast beef averages 40 calories, 1g fat and 40mg sodium per 28g (1oz) • Lean Black Forest ham averages 30 calories, 0.5g fat and 290mg sodium per 28g (1oz)

Choices to avoid

These choices have more fat, more calories and, in some cases, a lot more sodium, too: Mortadella averages 88 calories, 7.2g fat and 353mg sodium per 28g (1oz) • Pastrami and salt beef average 150 calories, 1.5g fat and 450mg sodium per 28g (1oz) • Genoa salami averages 110 calories, 9g fat and 520mg sodium per 28g (1oz) • Hard salami averages 104 calories, 8g fat and 560mg sodium per 28g (1oz)

Nutritional analysis
per 113g (4oz) roast beef on rye bread as pictured

332 calories, with 33 per cent from fat; **12.2g** fat, of which, **3.8g** saturated fat; **35.8g** protein; **95mg** cholesterol; **819mg** sodium; **2.3g** fibre

Vegetarian options

Versatile tofu is the protein-rich choice for vegetarians

Use 170g (6oz) tofu for a dinner that only takes minutes (for the recipe, *see page 173*).

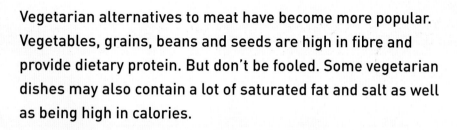

Vegetarian alternatives to meat have become more popular. Vegetables, grains, beans and seeds are high in fibre and provide dietary protein. But don't be fooled. Some vegetarian dishes may also contain a lot of saturated fat and salt as well as being high in calories.

A vegetarian red bean and cheese enchilada can be as high in fat and calories as a double hamburger with cheese. Deep-fried tofu served with a rich soy sauce can also be laden with fat and salt. Be warned.

Choices to savour

Dried or roasted nuts and seeds (such as sunflower or pumpkin) without added oil or salt average 180 calories per 28g (1oz) • Soft or firm tofu is high in protein and averages 130–250 calories per 170g (6oz) • Legumes (red beans, black beans, haricot beans, lentils) average 110–150 calories per 86–130g (3–4½oz) • Seitan, also known as wheat gluten and resembling meat in both appearance and taste, averages 210 calories per 57g (2oz) • Tahini, made from crushed sesame seeds, and with a creamy, nutty taste, averages 175 calories per 2 tbsp • Tempeh, used as a meat substitute in many dishes, averages 230 calories per 113g (4oz) • TVP (textured vegetable protein) has very little fat and averages 160 calories per 57g (2oz)

Choices to watch

Nuts and seeds that have been roasted in oil with added salt • Cream • Eggs *(see pages 66–67)* • Cheese *(see pages 64–65)* • Whole milk *(see pages 58–59)* • Salty sauces, such as soy sauce

Forewarned is forearmed

Some prepackaged vegetarian meals (mostly frozen) advertise themselves as 'wholesome and natural', but this doesn't always mean healthy. These meals might have an excessive amount of cheese and salt along with a very high calorie count.

Nutritional analysis
per 170g (6oz) tofu portion as pictured

132 calories, with 56 per cent from fat; **8.2g** fat, of which, **1.2g** saturated fat; **13.7g** protein; **0mg** cholesterol; **12mg** sodium; **0.6g** fibre
(see page 178 for nutritional analysis of whole plate)

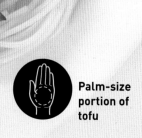

Palm-size portion of tofu

fish and shellfish

Really fresh fish and shellfish are a treat. What is more, they are the original fast foods, taking only minutes to cook. And if that weren't enough, they are low in unhealthy saturated fat and rich in omega-3 fatty acids, which have been proved to protect us from heart disease. But, as with all foods, it's the portion size that counts and the way that you prepare them. So, whether your favourite is white-fleshed sole, heart-healthy salmon or plump and juicy prawns, read the following pages to discover the perfect portion sizes and the healthiest cooking tips around. To discover how to incorporate fish and shellfish in your perfect portion plan on a regular basis, see my Seven-Day Eating Plan on pages 160–180.

White fish

All fish contain omega-3 fatty acids. White, non-oily, fish has fewer than others but still should be enjoyed regularly. Skip the Hollandaise and butter; instead try the suggestions here for white-fish dinners that are a healthy treat.

How much can I eat?

Plan on a 170g (6oz) portion of uncooked fish (142g/5oz cooked), which averages 168 calories with 8–19 per cent from fat, depending on the variety.

Choices to savour

This large group of fish includes the following: Cod • Flatfish (plaice or sole) • Grey mullet • Grouper • Haddock • Hake • Halibut • John Dory • Mahi-mahi • Monkfish • Orange roughy • Perch • Red mullet • Red snapper • Sea bass • Sea bream • Sea trout • Turbot • Yellowfin or albacore tuna

Healthy ways to enjoy

It goes without saying that you should not eat your fish deep-fried or covered in a thick layer of batter or breadcrumbs. Nor should you choose a rich, buttery sauce. So how can you make your fish extra tasty without piling on the calories and fat? Try these tempting suggestions:
• Sauté in 2 tsp olive or rapeseed oil and top with 2 tbsp tomato or fruit salsa (e.g peach or mango) per person.
• Thread cubed fish on skewers, grill or barbecue, and serve with 1 tbsp bottled satay peanut sauce per person.
• Spray with olive oil spray. Bake, sauté or barbecue, and serve with a sauce made from 1 tbsp mayonnaise mixed with the juice of a fresh tomato.

Nutritional analysis
per 170g (6oz) sole portion as pictured

156 calories, with 12 per cent from fat; **2g** fat, of which, **0.5g** saturated fat; **32g** protein; **84mg** cholesterol; **138mg** sodium; **0g** fibre
(see page 176 for nutritional analysis of whole plate)

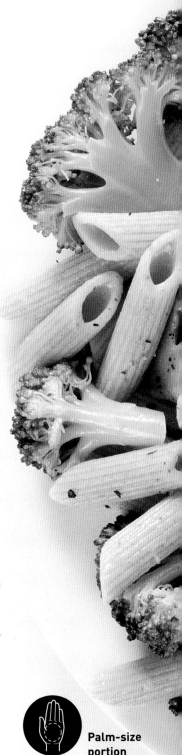

Palm-size
portion

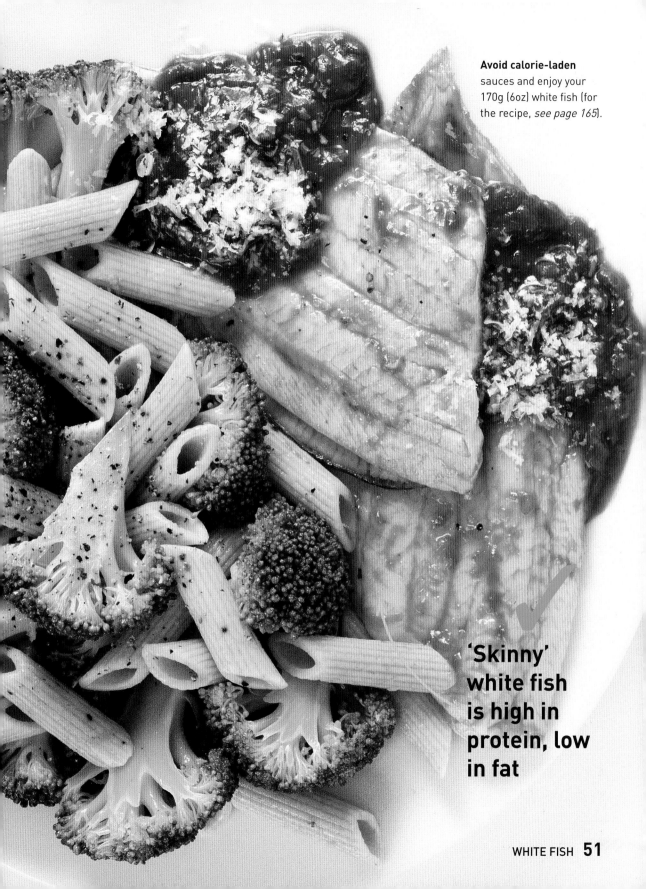

Avoid calorie-laden sauces and enjoy your 170g (6oz) white fish (for the recipe, *see page 165*).

'Skinny' white fish is high in protein, low in fat

Omega-3-rich fish

These fish are super-good for you as they contain even more omega-3 fatty acids than their white fish relatives. But, as with everything else, portion size counts. Eat too much and your waistline will most definitely expand.

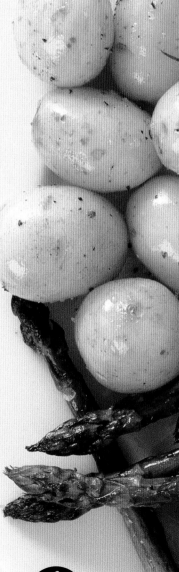

How much can I eat?
Plan on a 170g (6oz) portion of uncooked fish (142g/5oz cooked).

Choices to savour
The following 170g (6oz) portions of fish are the best sources of omega-3 fatty acids: Mackerel and sardines (both with about 360 calories with 50–60 per cent from fat) • Salmon, trout, herring, and bluefin tuna (all of which have about 250 calories with 30–50 per cent from fat)

Healthy ways to enjoy
Stay away from deep-fried fish or fish covered with a rich buttery sauce or a thick layer of batter or breadcrumbs. The healthiest ways to cook these fish are to barbecue, grill, poach or sauté them. They are so flavourful that they don't need sauces or seasoning. Just 1–2 tsp olive oil and salt and pepper will bring out their natural flavour. Alternatively, you can:
- Dip fish fillets in a bought Jamaican jerk or other spicy seasoning and sauté in 1 tsp olive or rapeseed oil per person.
- Top cooked fish with 3 tbsp tinned roasted red peppers and 6 chopped black olives per person.
- Spoon 1 tbsp chutney or relish per person on top.
- Serve cooked fish with a sauce of 1 tbsp mayonnaise mixed with 1 tsp horseradish per person.

Nutritional analysis
per 170g (6oz) salmon portion as pictured

240 calories, with 40 per cent from fat; **10.7g** fat, of which, **1.7g** saturated fat; **33.7g** protein; **96mg** cholesterol; **72mg** sodium; **0g** fibre
(see page 177 for nutritional analysis of whole plate)

Palm-size portion

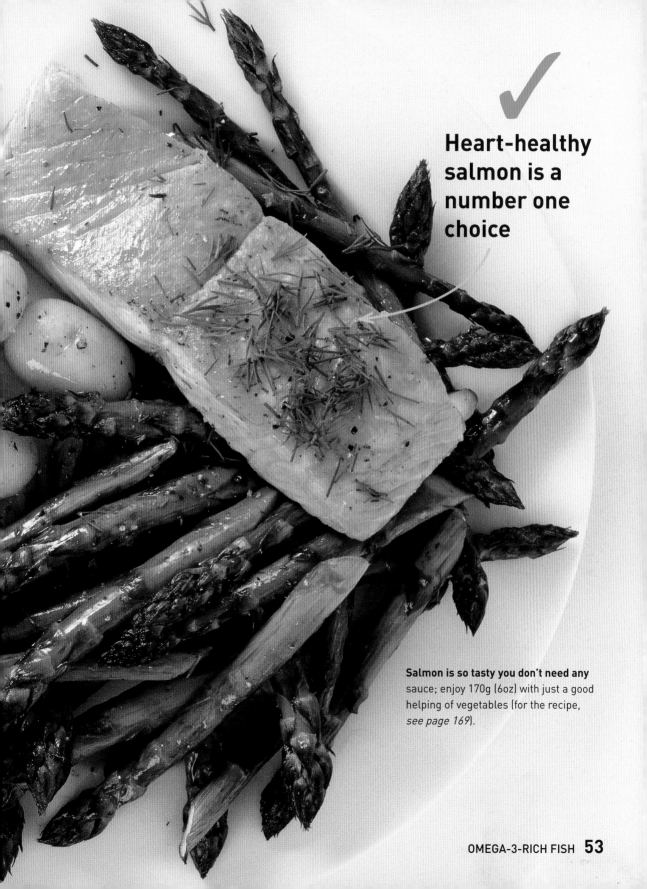

Heart-healthy salmon is a number one choice

Salmon is so tasty you don't need any sauce; enjoy 170g (6oz) with just a good helping of vegetables (for the recipe, *see page 169*).

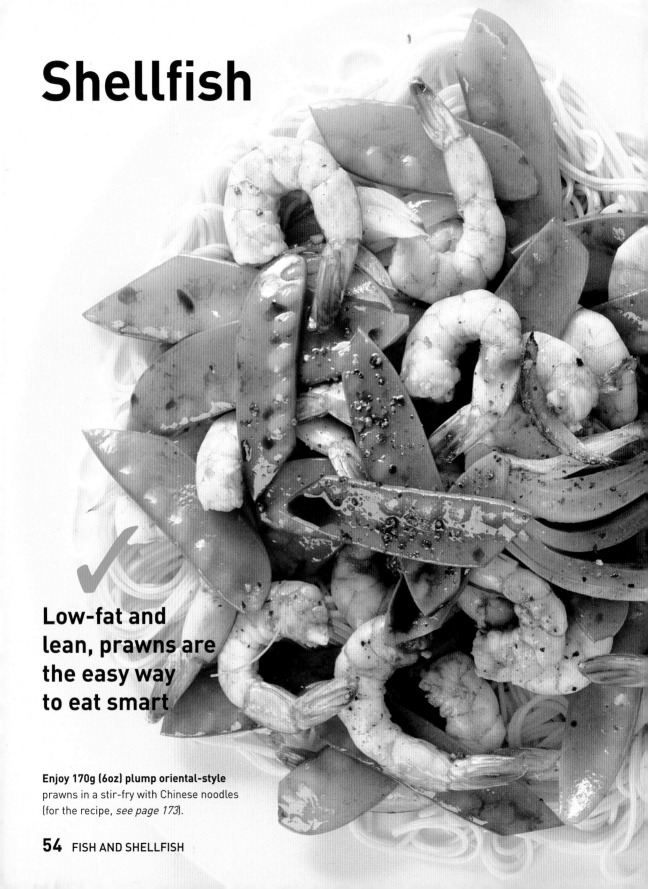

Shellfish

Low-fat and
lean, prawns are
the easy way
to eat smart

Enjoy 170g (6oz) plump oriental-style
prawns in a stir-fry with Chinese noodles
(for the recipe, *see page 173*).

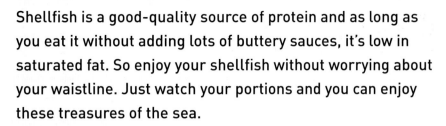

Shellfish is a good-quality source of protein and as long as you eat it without adding lots of buttery sauces, it's low in saturated fat. So enjoy your shellfish without worrying about your waistline. Just watch your portions and you can enjoy these treasures of the sea.

How much can I eat?
Plan on a 170g (6oz) portion of uncooked, shelled fish (142g/5oz cooked), which averages 155 calories with about 13 per cent from fat.

Choices to savour
There are plenty of different shellfish to enjoy. Choose from these according to your personal preferences: Clams • Crab • Crayfish • Lobster • Mussels • Octopus • Oysters • Prawns • Scallops • Squid

Choices to avoid
Shellfish in heavy sauces such as thermidor, au gratin, hollandaise, mornay • Deep-fried shellfish • Shellfish heavily coated with breadcrumbs • Shellfish with breadcrumb-based stuffing

Healthy ways to enjoy
• Lobster – steam or boil and serve with a sauce made by melting 1 tsp butter with 2 tsp rapeseed oil. Or, serve cold with a mayonnaise sauce made from 1 tbsp reduced-fat mayonnaise mixed with 1 tbsp fresh lemon or lime juice.
• Prawns – steam or boil, and serve with 2 tbsp of a tomato-based cocktail sauce. Or, sauté or stir-fry with vegetables.
• Crab – steam or boil, and serve cold, tossed with a sauce made from 1 tbsp reduced-fat mayonnaise and 1 tbsp ketchup.
• Mussels and clams – cook with carrots, celery, onion and a little white wine. Serve in their shells with the resulting sauce.

Nutritional analysis
per 170g (6oz) prawns portion as pictured

250 calories, with 35 per cent from fat; **18g** fat, of which, **7g** saturated fat; **35g** protein; **116mg** cholesterol; **94mg** sodium; **0g** fibre
(see page 178 for nutritional analysis of whole plate)

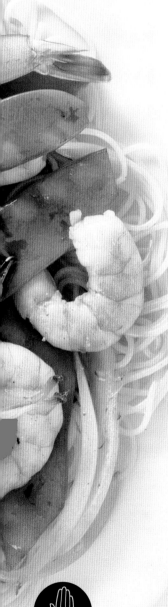

Palm-size portion

dairy

Dairy products contain protein, which helps us to feel full. Most importantly, though, they are the best food source of calcium. Get your daily requirement from eating three to four portions a day. They will help to keep your bones and teeth strong and healthy. Studies have also shown that calcium helps reduce the risk of high blood pressure and colon cancer. Take care, though. Products made from milk that have little or no calcium are cream cheese, cream and butter – and these are high in calories, too. The following pages give you a perfect portion look at how you can add dairy-rich calcium to your day without breaking your fat–calorie bank. To discover how to incorporate dairy foods in your perfect portion plan on a regular basis, see my Seven-Day Eating Plan on pages 160–180.

Milk and yogurt

Milk and yogurt are great ways to get your three to four dairy portions a day. They are fortified with vitamins, which means they're chock-full of health. But danger lies ahead if you choose whole milk. Your choice should be skimmed or semi-skimmed milk instead.

Yogurt can be a tricky choice, too. The supermarket aisles are filled with a bewildering array of pots and trays made with full-fat yogurt. These often have sugar, granola and even chocolate-covered cereal added to the yogurt. Ingredients like these not only add calories, but replace some of the nutrient-rich yogurt that would otherwise be there. You could find yourself eating 260 calories with extra saturated fat at the expense of the protein, calcium and vitamins in the 'missing' yogurt. By contrast, a 227g (8oz) fat-free, fruit-flavoured yogurt would weigh in at 80–100 calories.

How much can I have?

Plan on having 237ml (8fl oz) of skimmed milk or 227g (8oz) fat-free yogurt as one portion. If you are lactose-intolerant, 237ml (8fl oz) of calcium-fortified, fat-free or low-fat soya milk is a good alternative.

Make mine a 237ml (8fl oz) glass of skimmed milk

Drinking skimmed milk means you won't be having too much saturated fat in your daily diet.

Nutritional analysis

per 237ml (8fl oz) skimmed milk portion as pictured

86 calories with 5 per cent from fat; **0.4g** fat, of which, **0.3g** saturated fat; **8.4g** protein; **5mg** cholesterol; **127mg** sodium; **0g** fibre

Choices to savour
Make these your favourites: Skimmed or semi-skimmed milk • A 227g (8oz) carton of fat-free, low-sugar yogurt, which contains between 80 and 100 calories, depending on the brand

Choices to watch
Whole milk • Flavoured milk • Whole-milk yogurt • Granola-topped yogurt • Sweetened fruit yogurt • Sweetened yogurt drinks • Milk-based desserts such as chocolate pudding

Frozen yogurt – the unexpected dangers
Frozen yogurt is not the road to take if you want to put dairy foods on your list. It's good for a treat if you stick to just 72g (2¾oz). Yes, it has calcium, but very little compared with regular, fat-free yogurt, and many frozen yogurts are filled with sugar or saturated fat. A typical 186g (6½oz) serving of sugar-free, fat-free frozen yogurt has about 200 calories; a typical 174g (6¼oz) serving of low-fat frozen yogurt with sugar has about 220 calories.

Plain, fat-free, low-sugar yogurt can be dressed up with fresh fruit to make a healthy breakfast.

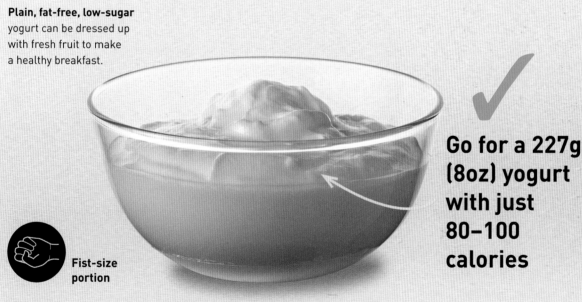

Fist-size portion

Go for a 227g (8oz) yogurt with just 80–100 calories

Nutritional analysis
per 227g (8oz) plain, fat-free, low-sugar yogurt portion as pictured

98 calories with 4 per cent from fat; **0.4g** fat, of which, **0.3g** saturated fat; **8.8g** protein; **5mg** cholesterol; **134mg** sodium; **0g** fibre

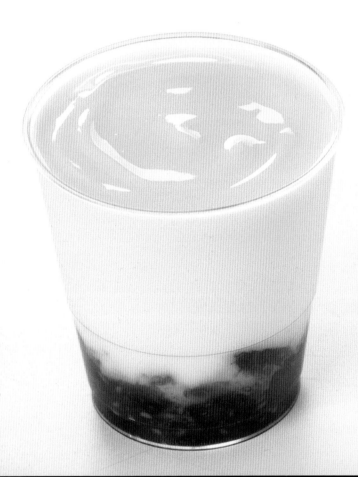

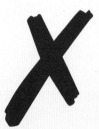

**On sale
everywhere for**

260

calories

oversize portion

You may think yogurt is a healthy choice, but eat one of the many 227g (8oz) yogurts with fruit on the bottom that are on sale everywhere, and you'll be getting about 260 calories. The reason? Most contain sugar and fat. And yogurts with sugary, cereal, chocolate or toffee toppings are another culprit. These can be 240 calories and up. All of these are more than double the calories of fruit-flavoured, fat-free yogurt.

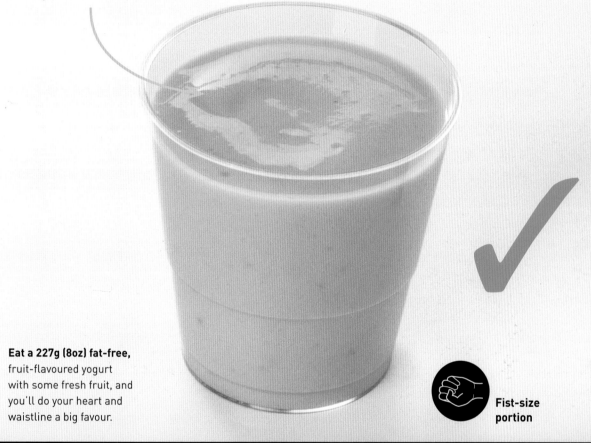

No fat and no sugar
for just 100 calories

Eat a 227g (8oz) fat-free,
fruit-flavoured yogurt
with some fresh fruit, and
you'll do your heart and
waistline a big favour.

**Fist-size
portion**

perfect portion

Your best yogurt bet is a 227g (8oz) fat-free,
fruit-flavoured yogurt made with sugar
substitute. That way you'll only be getting
100 calories. Look for yogurt brands that
contain active cultures. These aid in digestion.
Try mixing yogurt with bran cereal at breakfast
as an alternative to skimmed milk. Eat a 227g
(8oz) fat-free carton as a dessert at lunch or
as a mid-afternoon snack.

Nutritional analysis
per 227g (8oz) fat-free yogurt as pictured

98 calories; **0.4g** fat, of which, **0.3g** saturated
fat; **8.8g** protein; **5mg** cholesterol; **134mg**
sodium; **0g** fibre

Dairy-based toppings

Butter, mayonnaise and cream add great flavour to sandwiches, meats and many recipes. In addition, they contain nutrients although, unlike milk, cheese and yogurt, they have little or no calcium. But the main problem with them is that they also contain unhealthy fat as well as lots of calories. A thick layer of butter spread on your bread can add 204 calories and 23g of fat, while five tablespoons of mayo in that sandwich add a hefty 297 calories and 33g of fat.

How much can I eat?

There's no need to eliminate fats and oils from your food completely – in fact we need them for a balanced diet. Simply think teaspoons instead of tablespoons. And when it comes to your butter portion, one teaspoon is what you should be aiming for. Avoid using margarines or spreads containing trans fats as a replacement for dairy-based spreads. Trans fat is liquid fat that has been altered by partial hydrogenation to turn it into solids that are similar to saturated fats. Watch out for food labels with the words 'trans fats' or 'partially hydrogenated'.

Aim to limit your butter to 1 tsp or choose a butter substitute without trans fat instead.

Healthy ways to enjoy

- Mix 1 tsp butter with 2 tsp rapeseed oil per person for butter flavour with less saturated fat on your fish or cooked vegetables.
- Looking for the satisfying flavour of real mayonnaise? Mix the 'real thing' with other ingredients to spread its flavour while cutting the fat. For example, mix 1/2 tbsp mayonnaise with 1/2 tbsp fat-free yogurt per person.
- 1 tbsp mayonnaise mixed with 1 tbsp fresh lime or lemon juice per person will dress a chicken salad, fish salad, vegetable salad, potato salad or coleslaw.
- Add variety to the above mayonnaise toppings by adding one of the following: 1 tbsp prepared horseradish; 1 tbsp fresh chopped herbs; 45g (1½oz) chopped fresh tomatoes; 2 tsp curry powder; 1 tbsp chopped fresh ginger; 1 tbsp honey mustard; 1 tbsp sweet pickle.
- Real cream gives flavour and texture to many dishes. You should use 1 tbsp per person.
- Choose light or low-fat mayonnaise instead of real mayonnaise.

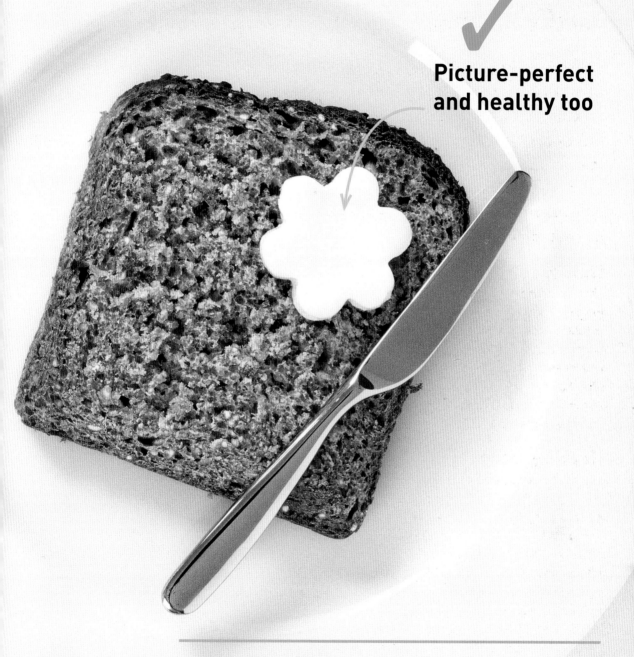

Picture-perfect and healthy too

Nutritional analysis

per 1 tsp butter on 28g (1oz) wholemeal bread as pictured

103 calories with 44 per cent from fat; **5g** fat, of which, **2.7g** saturated fat; **2.8g** protein; **10mg** cholesterol; **187mg** sodium; **1.9g** fibre

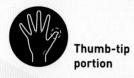

Thumb-tip portion

Cheese

A perfect portion of grated reduced-fat Cheddar cheese has 74–98 calories with 3–4g fat.

Cupped-hand portion

Choose just one 43–57g (1½–2oz) portion of reduced-fat cheese for a healthy choice

A perfect portion of reduced-fat Cheddar cheese has 74–98 calories with 3–4g fat.

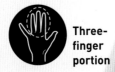

Three-finger portion

A perfect portion of
reduced-fat Emmenthal
cheese has 75–100
calories with 2.1–2.8g fat.

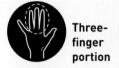

**Three-
finger
portion**

Cheese finds its way into your food in all kinds of ways –
from the cheese on your pizza, to the melted cheese on
your cheeseburger and, of course, in your macaroni cheese.
Mature Cheddar cheese adds a tasty sparkle to an omelette,
while the nutty flavour of French Brie adds a special touch
to a baguette sandwich. But is cheese a good thing?

All cheeses are packed with nutrition and especially with calcium, so they
can be a valued part of your portion plan. But, it's important to watch the
portions. You can savour the flavours and textures of cheese, guilt-free,
if you follow these guidelines.

How much can I eat?

Plan on 43–57g (1½–2oz) reduced-fat cheese as a portion.

Choices to savour

Reduced-fat cheese • Reduced-fat cream cheese • Reduced-fat cottage
cheese • Part-skimmed-milk ricotta cheese

Choices to watch

Full-fat cheeses • Full-fat cheese spreads • Cheese toppings • Full-fat
cream cheese • Cheese sauces and soups

Cheese alert

Select reduced-fat cheese over full-fat cheese to lower your calorie and
fat intake. Compare 43g (1½oz) of the following full-fat cheeses to those
reduced-fat cheeses pictured on the left and see the difference: full-fat
Cheddar cheese has 171 calories with 14.1g fat; full-fat Emmenthal has
162 calories with 11.9g fat.

Watch the tempting cheese challenges when you go out to eat or you'll
quickly break your calorie bank:

- Potato skins loaded with cheese and bacon are a popular appetizer but just
  100g (3¾oz) will give you a sixth of your recommended daily fat allowance.
- Do you enjoy that eat-out favourite of fried Camembert cheese and
  redcurrant jelly? Beware; it can add 264 calories and 17.6g of fat for
  a 57g (2oz) portion.
- Nachos with melted cheese can be yet another calorie disaster. One
  portion with 12–16 nachos, cheese and jalapeño peppers weighs in at
  over 1200 calories – that's almost an entire day's worth!

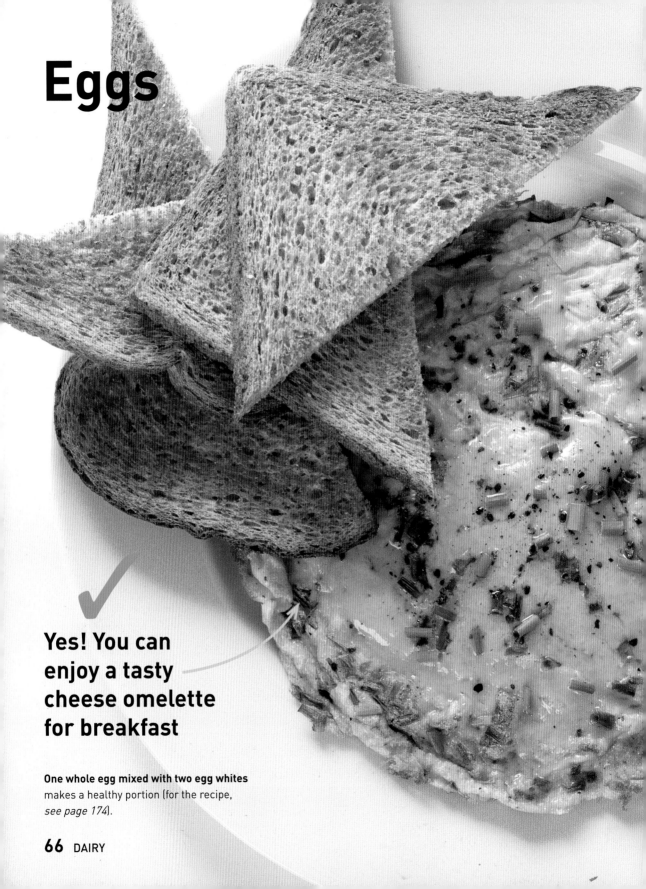

Eggs

✔

Yes! You can enjoy a tasty cheese omelette for breakfast

One whole egg mixed with two egg whites makes a healthy portion (for the recipe, *see page 174*).

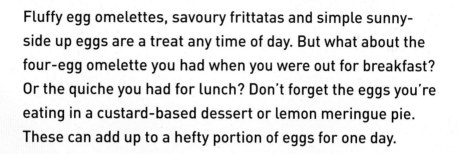

Fluffy egg omelettes, savoury frittatas and simple sunny-side up eggs are a treat any time of day. But what about the four-egg omelette you had when you were out for breakfast? Or the quiche you had for lunch? Don't forget the eggs you're eating in a custard-based dessert or lemon meringue pie. These can add up to a hefty portion of eggs for one day.

So what should you be eating? Basically, eggs are an excellent and inexpensive source of protein. The bacon and sausage you have with the omelette, or the sugar you have as part of the custard dessert are the real culprits here.

How much can I eat?

Enjoy your eggs and plan on one egg and two egg whites or two eggs as a portion.

Choices to avoid

You need to be on the alert to avoid eating lots of extra eggs each day without realizing it and to ensure that you eat eggs that have been prepared in a healthy way. These are the potential pitfalls: Hidden eggs in quiches, cakes and desserts • Omelettes made with more than two eggs • Eggs fried in butter, bacon or sausage fat • The sausage and bacon that often goes with the eggs • The sugar that's part of egg-based desserts

The latest news about eggs and cholesterol

Eggs have turned the corner. For many years eggs were thought to increase cholesterol levels. Today, studies have shown that people on a low-fat diet can eat one to two eggs a day without measurable changes in their blood cholesterol levels. If you prefer, you can enjoy your eggs *and* reduce your fat intake by mixing one whole egg with two egg whites as a portion.

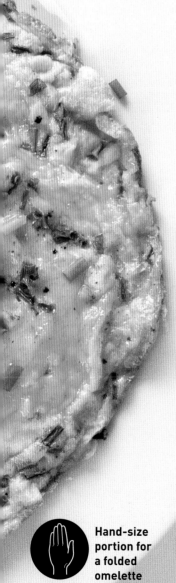

Hand-size portion for a folded omelette

Nutritional analysis
per 1 whole egg + 2 egg-white cheese omelette portion

174 calories, with 54 per cent from fat; **10.5g** fat, of which, **2.8g** saturated fat; **16.7g** protein; **216mg** cholesterol; **158mg** sodium; **1.7g** fibre
(see page 178 for nutritional analysis of whole breakfast)

vegetables and fruit

Eat your vegetables! This is a phrase we've all heard since childhood – even when our parents might not have been eating theirs. Well, they were right. We should be eating vegetables – and fruits, too. Both are important sources of nutrients and can help ward off heart disease and strokes.

What is more, they help control blood pressure and cholesterol, and may help to prevent some types of cancer. They are also high in fibre and can protect us from diverticulitis. Read the following pages to find your perfect portions of these invaluable foods. You'll quickly find how right your parents were.

To discover how to incorporate vegetables and fruit in your perfect portion plan on a regular basis, see my Seven-Day Eating Plan on pages 160–180.

No-worry vegetables

You know that vegetables are good for you, but how many meals do you eat with nothing green, or even red, orange or yellow on your plate? Now's the time to put matters right. Eating no-worry, low-calorie vegetables gives you extra nutrients and helps to fill you up.

How much can I eat?

The Food Standards Agency recommends we eat a minimum of five portions of vegetables and fruit a day (our 'Five a Day'), or a total of 400g (14oz). No-worry vegetables should form part of that. I recommend you eat 224–600g (8–21½oz) uncooked no-worry vegetables a day, but 112–300g (4–10¾oz) per meal is even better. If you like, you can drink a 237ml (8fl oz) glass of low-salt tomato or vegetable juice instead of a 56–150g (2–5½oz) serving of vegetables.

Eat 142g (5oz) per portion for tip-top health

Put something green on your plate with a 142g (5oz) portion of broccoli and only 50 calories.

Two-fist portion

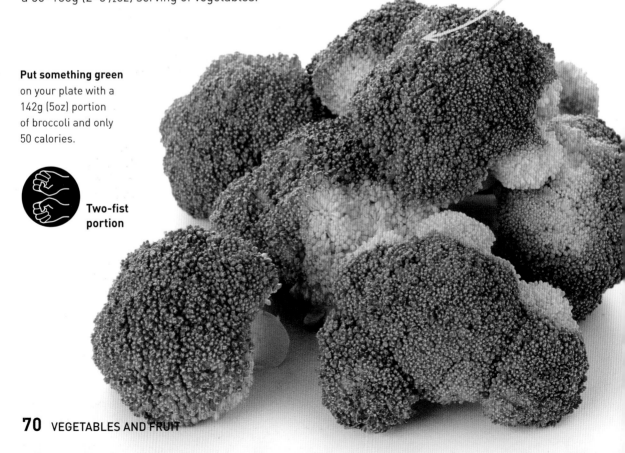

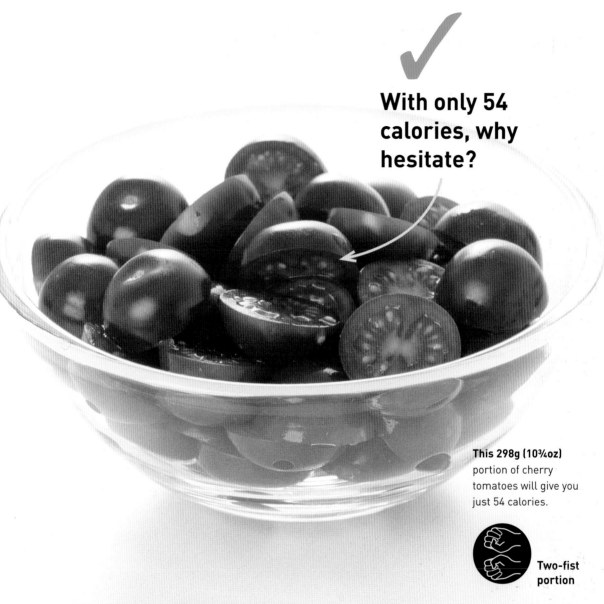

✓

With only 54 calories, why hesitate?

This 298g (10¾oz) portion of cherry tomatoes will give you just 54 calories.

Two-fist portion

Choices to savour

Any combination of these no-worry vegetables will help you achieve your vegetable portion goal: Acorn squash • Artichokes • Asparagus • Aubergines • Bean sprouts • Bok choy • Broccoli • Brussels sprouts • Butternut squash • Carrots • Cauliflower • Celery • Chinese cabbage • Courgettes • Cucumbers • Garlic • Green beans • Green, red and yellow peppers • Kale • Kohlrabi • Lettuce (all types) • Mushrooms • Okra • Onions • Pumpkin • Red cabbage • Runner beans • Spaghetti squash • Spinach • Spring greens • Tomatoes • White cabbage • Yellow squash

Vegetables to watch

All vegetables are good for us, but not all vegetables were born equal. Portions for starchy vegetables – my 'vegetables to watch' – are different from other vegetables. They should be eaten in moderation but should still form part of your minimum 'Five a Day' fruit and vegetable portions.

These starchy vegetables are good, nutritional carbohydrates and are an important part of our everyday meal plan, but they should be eaten in smaller quantities than other vegetables because they are high in calories and carbohydrates.

How much can I eat?
Plan on 67–73g (2½–2¾oz) uncooked per portion for the following vegetables:
- Sweetcorn
- Peas
- Potatoes
- Sweet potatoes
- Yams
- Broad beans
- Parsnips

Eat starchy vegetables in smaller portions

Sweet potato is always a favourite – 67g (2½oz) has 56 calories.

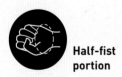

Half-fist portion

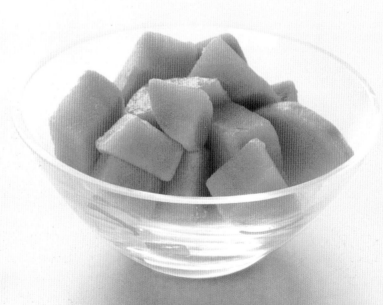

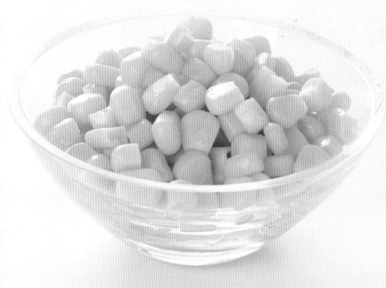

A 72g (2¾oz) portion of sweetcorn will give you 66 calories.

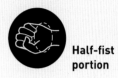

Half-fist portion

Healthy ways to enjoy

- The best way to prepare these vegetables is to boil, steam or – if you are in a hurry as they take time to cook – microwave them.
- Use frozen vegetables to shorten cooking and peeling time.
- If using tinned vegetables, look for 'no salt added' on the label.
- Purée these vegetables and use to thicken soups, gravies and stews instead of flour. This adds flavour, nutrients and texture to your dish.
- Don't serve with buttery, creamy sauces.
- Use these vegetables as a filling alternative to pasta and rice.

Eat a 73g (2¾oz) portion of peas for 56 calories.

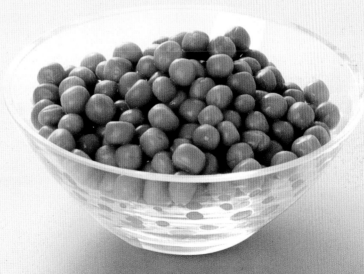

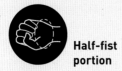

Half-fist portion

Potatoes

✓

Mashed potatoes need not give you more than 207 calories per 113g (4oz) portion.

Cupped-hand portion

Choose one of these for part of a healthy meal

✓

Waxy potatoes without butter total around 100 calories per 113g (4oz) portion.

Cupped-hand portion

In 1960, Americans consumed an average of 37 kilograms (81lb) of fresh potatoes and 1.8 kilograms (4lb) of frozen chips per year. By 2000, that had risen to about 68 kilograms (150lb) of fresh potatoes and 14 kilograms (30lb) of frozen chips. All that potato ends up on our waistlines...

How much can I eat?

Plan on a portion size of 113–170g (4–6oz) cooked potato. If you are physically active for an hour a day, you can safely increase that amount to 227g (8oz).

Healthy ways to enjoy

Here are some tips on how you can love your potatoes and not break the portion and calorie bank:

- Add other vegetables to stretch your portion size.
- Use waxy potatoes such as Pink Fir Apple, Charlotte or Cara. These types need less fat to make them moist and flavourful than a floury potato such as King Edward.
- Boiled new potatoes are so sweet they only need a little oil, salt and pepper. Add chives or parsley for extra flavour and colour.
- Enjoy roasted rosemary potatoes. Here's how. Toss potato cubes in a little olive oil, sprinkle with fresh rosemary, salt and pepper, and bake for 30–40 minutes at 200°C (400°F/Gas 6).
- Sauté sliced potatoes in fat-free, low-sodium chicken stock to cover, with 1 tbsp rapeseed oil, until the potatoes are tender and the stock is absorbed.

Mashed potato tricks

Mashed potatoes are a favourite but if you make them with butter and cream, they will add loads of fat and calories. Enjoy your mashed potatoes by following these cooking tips for a 113g (4oz) potato portion:

- Use 118ml (4fl oz) skimmed milk with about 1 tsp butter for flavour and 1 tsp rapeseed oil.
- Mash the potato using some of the cooking water with a little garlic and olive oil instead of cream or milk and butter.
- Mix 59ml (2fl oz) buttermilk into the mashed potato instead of cream or milk and butter, and sprinkle with chives.
- Boil or microwave 113g (4oz) vegetables (cauliflower, fennel, celery), add to the cooked potatoes and mash together using one of the mashed potato tricks above.

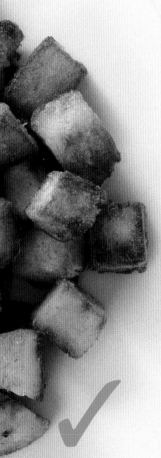

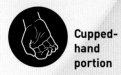

Sauté your potatoes in rapeseed or olive oil for 170 calories per 113g (4oz) portion.

Cupped-hand portion

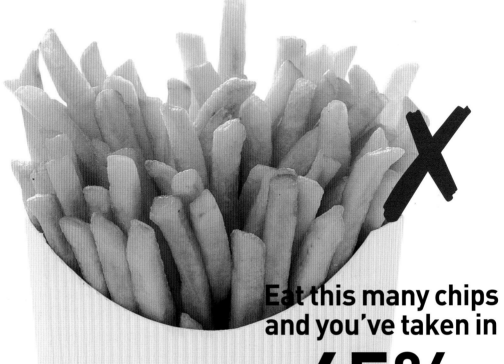

Eat this many chips and you've taken in

45%

of your daily calories

oversize portion

Do you have any idea by how much portions of chips have grown in size? Today's average 198g (7oz) serving has about 610 calories. This compares to a 210-calorie portion that was the norm twenty years ago. That means a huge, three-fold increase. And it makes for huge people, too. A 73kg (160lb) person would need to walk at a leisurely pace for 1 hour and 10 minutes to use up all those calories.

Do the maths! About 20 chips = 1 portion

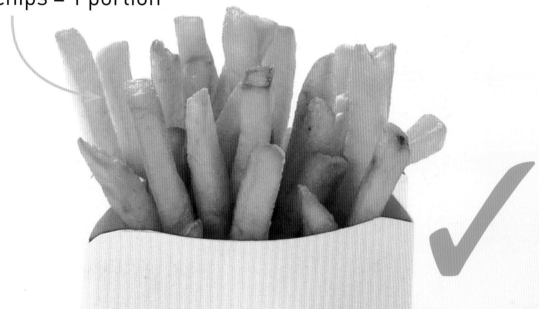

Make your portion of chips about 85g (3oz) fried in liquid corn or rapeseed oil. Oven-baked are healthier (*see below*).

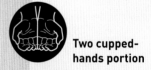

Two cupped-hands portion

perfect portion

For oven-baked chips, preheat the oven to 230°C (450°F/Gas 8) and line a baking sheet with foil. Brush the foil with 1 tbsp rapeseed oil. Peel then cut 113g (4oz) potatoes into strips and lay on the baking sheet. Toss in the oil to make sure all sides are covered. Sprinkle lightly with salt. Bake on the middle shelf of the oven for 15 minutes, then turn the potatoes over, and bake for a further 15 minutes or until they are crisp.

Nutritional analysis
per 85g (3oz) portion of chips as pictured

210 calories with 58 per cent fat; **13.6g** fat, of which, **1.8g** saturated fat; **2.4g** protein; **20.5g** carbohydrate; **0mg** cholesterol; **6mg** sodium; **1.5g** fibre

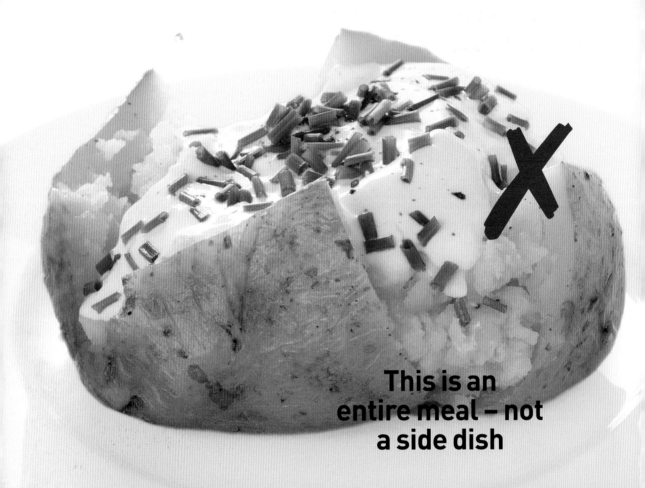

This is an entire meal – not a side dish

oversize portion

The problem with baked potatoes isn't the potato but the topping. If you eat the enormous 340g (12oz) baked potato shown here, with all that butter and soured cream, you'll be getting 578 calories. That's the amount of calories you should have for an entire meal, not for a side dish. This is a typical restaurant serving size. And watch out for that baked potato with vegetables and a thick cheese sauce that's often served for lunch.

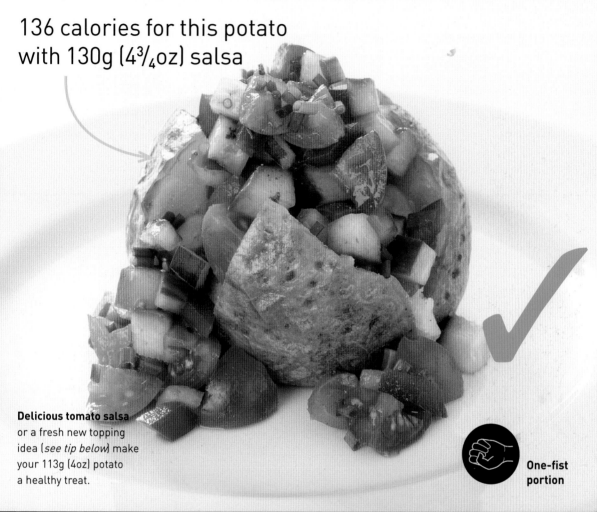

136 calories for this potato with 130g (4¾oz) salsa

Delicious tomato salsa or a fresh new topping idea (*see tip below*) make your 113g (4oz) potato a healthy treat.

One-fist portion

perfect portion

Try these other delicious potato topping ideas on a 113g (4oz) potato:
• 1 tbsp reduced-fat soured cream mixed with 1 tbsp plain fat-free yogurt and topped with chopped chives
• 2 tbsp fat-free yogurt, mixed with 2 tsp wholegrain mustard and 2 tbsp chopped spring onions
• Microwave 35g (1¼oz) sliced mushrooms with 1 tsp olive oil and add chopped parsley

Nutritional analysis
per 113g (4oz) baked potato with salsa

136 calories with 2 per cent from fat; **0.4g** fat, of which, **0.1g** saturated fat; **4.4g** protein; **0mg** cholesterol; **563mg** sodium; **3.3g** fibre

Legumes

✓

Add some delicious crudités to turn 2 tbsp of houmus – made from chickpeas – into a tasty hors d'œuvres or a snack.

Eat healthy houmus and crudités for a tasty snack

Baked beans, black beans and rice, split-pea soup – all of these are comfort foods that many of us love. And what's more, these legumes are good for us, too, since they are packed with fibre and vegetable protein. It's easy to add legumes to your daily menu. Toss them in a salad, mix with brown rice, add them to wraps or blend them with spices into a pâté or spread. But remember, they are not good for you if you eat an entire plateful.

How much can I eat?

Count on 84–99g (3–3½oz, depending on variety) cooked legumes as a portion, which assumes that you will be adding them to other ingredients in a dish, rather than eating them on their own.

Choices to savour

The legumes are all healthy choices. Try: Black beans • Black-eyed beans • Butter beans • Cannellini beans • Chickpeas • Haricot beans • Kidney beans • Lentils • Pinto beans • Split peas • Good quality houmus – made from chickpeas – is available in most supermarkets. Keep some on hand for snacks. Just 2 tbsp are great with crudités or on crackers.

Cooking tips

Mostly you need to soak raw legumes overnight before you cook them. If you don't have time for this, use tinned beans instead. They have the same nutritional value as raw beans. Be sure to rinse and drain the beans. Lentils are one legume that do not need to be soaked. They take about 20 minutes to cook in boiling water.

Vegetarian choice

Legumes are a great source of protein for vegetarians. The vegetarian alternative dinners in my Seven-Day Eating Plan (*see pages 160–175*) give you ideas on how to substitute legumes in your meals.

Nutritional analysis
per 2 tbsp houmus and crudités as pictured

107 calories, with 28 per cent from fat; **3.3g** fat, of which, **0.5g** saturated fat; **4.2g** protein; **0mg** cholesterol; **194mg** sodium; **61.g** fibre

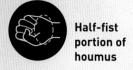

Half-fist portion of houmus

Salads

Green salads can form part of your minimum 'Five a Day' portions of vegetables and fruit. They have almost no calories and add good nutrients to a meal. Fill your plate with washed, ready-to-eat salad leaves and top with 113g (4oz) of grilled chicken or salmon for a quick lunch. Make it into a dinner by adding 170g (6oz) of chicken or salmon and serve with two slices of wholemeal bread or toss in 105g (3¾oz) cooked pasta.

Salad bars are a great way to eat your vegetables, and they're another alternative to chopping and slicing your own salads. But watch the dangers lurking there. Bacon bits, croûtons and salad dressings can quickly break your calorie bank.

How much can I eat?
Measure 94–110g (3½–4oz) of greens per person and 1 tbsp dressing. You will be surprised at how well this coats the salad. Or, keep your portion of dressing on the side and dip the salad into it as you eat. But, of course, this is only a guide. In fact, you can eat as much salad as you like.

Choices to savour
Measure your 40–360g (1½–13oz) from any of these vegetables or salad leaves: Baby leaf spinach • Celery • Cos • Cucumber • Frisée • Herbs • Iceberg • Lamb's lettuce • Little gem • Mizuna • Onion • Peppers (red, green, yellow and orange) • Radicchio • Radishes • Red mustard • Red oak leaf • Rocket • Romaine • Ruby chard • Tomatoes

Choices to watch
When it comes to those delicious salad 'extras', beware of the calories you will be adding: 1 tbsp bacon bits adds 33 calories • 8g (¼oz) of croûtons adds 46 calories • 1 tbsp pecans adds 51 calories • 1 tbsp walnuts adds 46 calories • 1 tbsp crumbled reduced-fat cheese adds 30 calories • 34g (1¼oz) of chopped hard-boiled egg adds 53 calories • 5 olives add 22 calories • 5 anchovy fillets add 42 calories • 1 tbsp grated Parmesan adds 22 calories

Green salads can form part of your 'Five a Day' vegetable and fruit portions

Crispy salad leaves are a tasty way to eat your veg

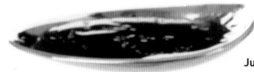

Just 1 tbsp of salad dressing will coat your portion of leaves. It only adds 72 calories and 8g fat.

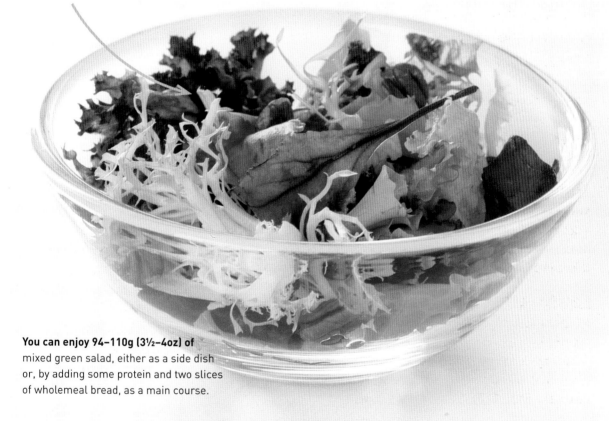

You can enjoy 94–110g (3½–4oz) of mixed green salad, either as a side dish or, by adding some protein and two slices of wholemeal bread, as a main course.

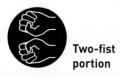

Two-fist portion

Nutritional analysis
per 94–110g (3½–4oz) mixed green salad as pictured

16 calories, with 17 per cent·from fat; **0.2g** fat, of which, **0g** saturated fat; **1.8g** protein; **2.7g** carbohydrate; **0mg** cholesterol; **8mg** sodium; **2g** fibre

Salad recipes

Potato salad and coleslaw are the perfect side dishes
to go with hamburgers and barbecued ribs, meat-filled
sandwiches or on a buffet table, but they can be unhealthy
choices. Try my recipes below for some healthy potato salad,
coleslaw and dressings that won't break the portion bank.

How much can I eat?

Measure 120g (4¼oz) coleslaw and 125g (4½oz) potato salad for a single
portion. If you include 92–101g (3¼–3¾oz) vegetables per person in your
potato salad, you may eat more and can measure a portion as 250g (9oz).

Mayonnaise-based coleslaw (Serves 1)

Mix 1 tbsp reduced-fat mayonnaise with 1 tbsp white vinegar, 1 tsp Dijon
mustard and ½ tsp sugar. Add salt and pepper to taste. Toss dressing over
70g (2½oz) shredded cabbage mixture, including any or all of the
following: sliced celery, sliced onions, sliced carrot or sliced spring onions.

Oil-and-vinegar-based coleslaw (Serves 1)

Add ½ tbsp prepared horseradish to 1 tbsp bottled oil-and-vinegar
dressing for 70g (2½oz) shredded cabbage mixture (*see above*).

Mayonnaise-based potato salad (Serves 1)

Mix 1 tbsp reduced-fat mayonnaise with 1 tbsp fat-free plain yogurt and
1 tsp Dijon mustard. Add chopped chives or other herbs if wished, and salt
and pepper to taste. Mix into 78g (2¾oz) boiled, cubed potatoes and add
some chopped celery, chopped green pepper or chopped onion to taste.

Oil-and-vinegar-based potato salad (Serves 1)

Mix 1 tbsp each white vinegar, Dijon mustard and cooking water from the
boiled potatoes with 1 tsp rapeseed oil. Mix with 78g (2¾oz) cubed potatoes
and some chopped celery, chopped green pepper or chopped onion to taste.

Make a meal of your potato salad (Serves 1)

Add 113g (4oz) roast chicken, seared tuna, cooked prawns or lean sausage
to your potato salad to turn a side dish into an entire meal.

Choose olive oil for a healthy heart

Use olive oil in small quantities to limit your calories and give you the monounsaturated fat you need in your diet.

Some quick salad dressings

Blue cheese dressing (I) (Serves 1)

Place 2 tsp red wine vinegar, 2 tsp olive oil and 14g (½ oz) crumbled blue cheese (Roquefort, Danish, Gorgonzola) in a small bowl or screw-top jar and mix well.

Blue cheese dressing (II) (Serves 1)

Place 14g (½ oz) crumbled blue cheese (Roquefort, Danish, Gorgonzola) and 1 tbsp low-fat bottled vinaigrette in a small bowl or screw-top jar and mix well.

Caesar dressing (Serves 1)

Add 1 rinsed, drained and finely chopped anchovy fillet to 1½ tbsp olive-oil-and-vinegar dressing in a bowl and mix well.

Vinaigrette dressing (Serves 1)

Place 1 tsp Dijon mustard and 1 tsp red wine vinegar in a bowl and mix together. Whisk in 2 tsp rapeseed or olive oil and add salt and pepper to taste.

Vinaigrette variations

Vinaigrette is a favourite, but it's nice to have a change. Try these variations:

* Add 1 small garlic clove, peeled and crushed
* Add 2 tsp chopped fresh herbs (e.g. parsley, chives, coriander, mint) or ½ tsp dried herbs
* Add 1 tbsp chopped fresh basil
* Add 1 tsp prepared horseradish
* Add 2 tsp finely chopped red onion
* Add 1 tsp peeled and grated fresh ginger
* Add 1 tsp low-sodium soya sauce

Oils

Monounsaturated and polyunsaturated oils are essential to good health. So what should we eat? Think in terms of 1 tsp (40 calories) when using them. Olive and rapeseed oil are the best sources of monounsaturated fat, while safflower, soya bean and sunflower oil are considered polyunsaturated. These are the 'right fats'. Beware though, palm and coconut oil are high in saturated fat and should be avoided.

Fruit

Displays of fruit in the produce department always make my mouth water but the best part is that fruits are also good for us and should form part of our minimum 'Five a Day' portions of fruit and vegetables. Fruit is filled with fibre and a variety of nutrients, which is great, but it also contains natural sugar. You should watch your intake to avoid adding too many sugar-laden calories to your diet.

Citrus fruits (oranges, grapefruits and tangerines) are packed with vitamin C. Bananas contain the essential mineral potassium as well as vitamin B6 and fibre. Pears and apples are loaded with about 4g fibre and if you leave the skin on, you will get extra. The tropical fruits – mango and papaya – are rich in fibre, vitamin C and carotinoids, which help the body maintain a strong immune system.

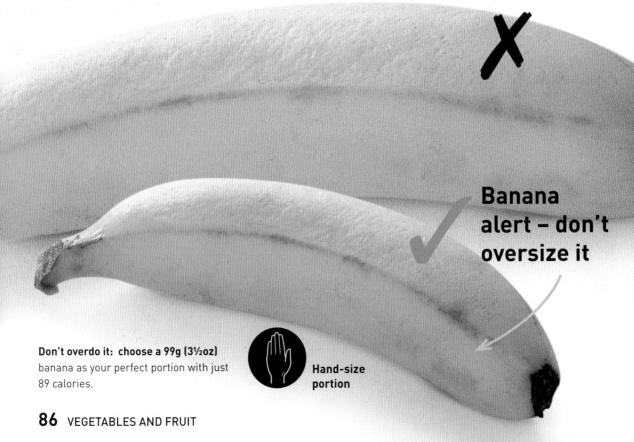

Banana alert – don't oversize it

Don't overdo it: choose a 99g (3½oz) banana as your perfect portion with just 89 calories.

Hand-size portion

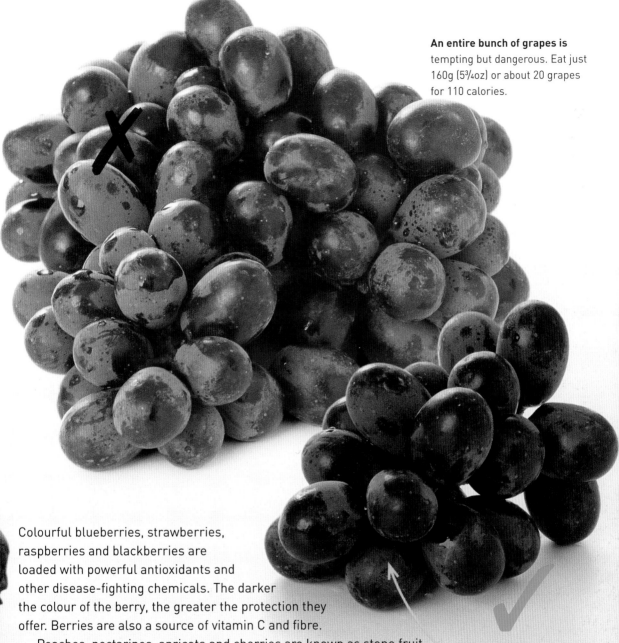

An entire bunch of grapes is tempting but dangerous. Eat just 160g (5¾oz) or about 20 grapes for 110 calories.

Colourful blueberries, strawberries, raspberries and blackberries are loaded with powerful antioxidants and other disease-fighting chemicals. The darker the colour of the berry, the greater the protection they offer. Berries are also a source of vitamin C and fibre.

Peaches, nectarines, apricots and cherries are known as stone fruit due to the large hard stone pit in the middle. These fruits also contain vitamin E, which is difficult to find in fat-free foods. In addition, apricots contain beta-carotene, which the body converts to vitamin A for healthy eyes, skin and mucous membranes.

When it comes to the different melons, cantaloupe, honeydew and watermelon are all low in calories and packed with vitamin C, folate and potassium. Cantaloupe is the most nutritious because of its concentrated beta-carotene content. Beta-carotene, which is also thought to reduce the

Twenty grapes are perfect

Cupped-hand portion

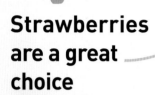

Strawberries are a great choice

Fist-size portion

Make 144g (5oz) of strawberries
part of your perfect portion plan for
only 45 calories.

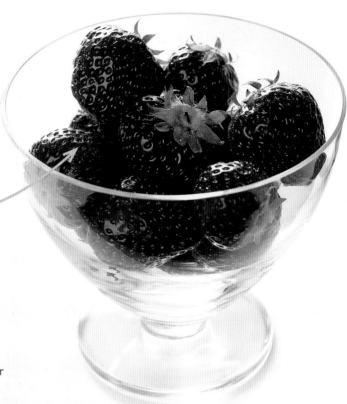

risk of chronic diseases, gives cantaloupe its orange colour. Watermelon contains lycopene, a cancer-fighting carotenoid.

How much can I eat?

As part of your 'Five a Day', I recommend you eat a daily 160–400g (5³/₄–14oz) of fruit. It's best to eat the whole fruit rather than just drink fruit juice, which doesn't contain any fibre and doesn't leave you feeling full.

Choices to savour

It's best to eat a variety of fruits but beware, as many fruits have ballooned in size. Measure a portion of these fruits to help you reach your target 160–400g (5³/₄–14oz) of fruit a day: Apples – one small (about 106g/3³/₄oz) • Apricots – four medium (about 155g/5¹/₂oz) • Bananas – one 20cm (8in) (about 118g/4¹/₄oz) • Blackberries, 145g (5oz) • Blueberries, 145g (5oz) • Cantaloupe melon, cubed, 160g (5³/₄oz) • Cherries, with stones, 117g (4oz) • Figs – four fresh (about 200g/7oz) • Grapefruit – one 10cm (4in) diameter (about 247g/9oz) • Grapes – about twenty (about 160g/5³/₄oz) • Honeydew melon, cubed, 170g (6oz) • Kiwis – 2 small (about 133g/4³/₄oz) • Mangoes – one medium (about 166g/6oz) • Nectarines – one medium (about 138g/4³/₄oz) • Oranges – one large (about 180g/6¹/₂oz) • Papaya, cubed,

140g (5oz) • Peaches – one medium (about 170g/6oz) • Pears – one medium (about 165g/6oz) • Pineapple, cubed, 155g (5¹/₂oz) • Plums – two large (about 165g/6oz) • Raspberries, 123g (4¹/₂oz) • Strawberries, whole, 144g (5oz) • Tangerines – two (about 196g/7oz) • Watermelon, cubed, 152g (5¹/₂oz)

Dried fruits

All dried fruits are high in calories and contain a lot of sugar. Plan on only 33g–41g (1–1¹/₂oz) per portion of them. They should be counted as part of your 160–400g (5³/₄–14oz) of fruit a day.

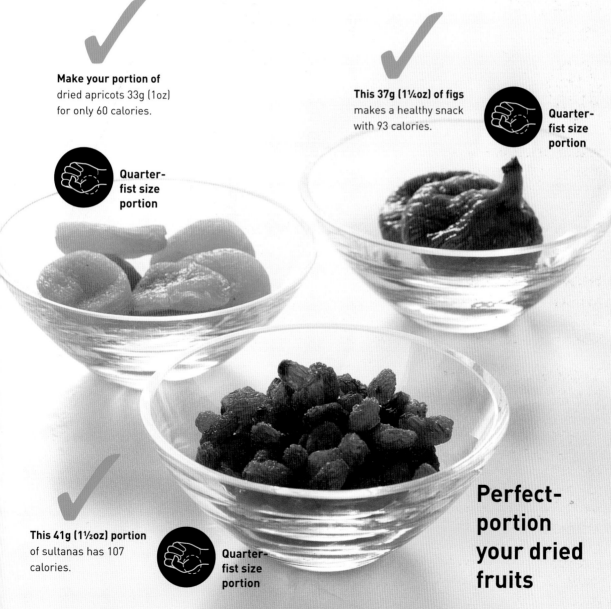

Make your portion of dried apricots 33g (1oz) for only 60 calories.

This 37g (1¼oz) of figs makes a healthy snack with 93 calories.

Quarter-fist size portion

Quarter-fist size portion

This 41g (1½oz) portion of sultanas has 107 calories.

Quarter-fist size portion

Perfect-portion your dried fruits

This 355ml (12fl oz) glass of orange juice contains

168

sugar-packed calories

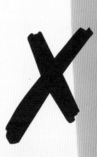

oversize portion

Orange juice has lots of vitamin C, but it's also full of sugar and has almost no fibre. Freshly squeezed orange juice is better, but you're drinking the equivalent of 5–6 oranges to get your 355ml (12fl oz) glass. The same is true for most other fruit juices as well. But the real danger zones are fruit drinks. Many of these are simply water, sugar and some fruit or fruit flavouring – just empty calories.

If you love your juice in the morning but are watching your waistline, start at the top of this list of recommendations per 177ml (6fl oz) portion and work your way down:

- Unsweetened grapefruit juice
  (71 calories, 17g carbohydrates)
- Fresh, unsweetened orange juice
  (84 calories, 19g carbohydrates)
- Unsweetened apple juice
  (90 calories, 22g carbohydrates)
- Unsweetened grape juice
  (96 calories, 24g carbohydrates)
- Unsweetened pineapple juice
  (102 calories, 24g carbohydrates)
- Prune juice
  (136 calories, 34g carbohydrates)

Try 177ml (6fl oz) of freshly squeezed orange juice for only 84 calories

perfect portion

Nutritional analysis
per 177ml (6fl oz) fresh orange juice portion

84 calories with 5 per cent from fat; **0.5g** fat, of which, **0.1g** saturated fat; **1.5g** protein; **0mg** cholesterol; **2mg** sodium; **0.4g** fibre

Freshly squeezed orange juice is good for you but lacks the fibre of the whole fruit.

grains

Grains are everywhere – in your bread, your bagels, your pastries, your breakfast cereal and your pizza. They're also what makes your pasta and noodles. Whole grains like whole-wheat pasta and brown rice contain the entire grain seed. They are complex carbohydrates that are slowly digested, so they are satisfying and help you feel full. Quickly digested, simple carbohydrates, such as white bread or white rice, often leave you with hunger pangs or cravings an hour after eating. Read the following pages to learn how much to eat for your perfect portion and how not to break your calorie bank by overloading those healthy grains with excess fat. To discover how to incorporate foods from the grains group in your perfect portion plan on a regular basis, see my Seven-Day Eating Plan on pages 160–180.

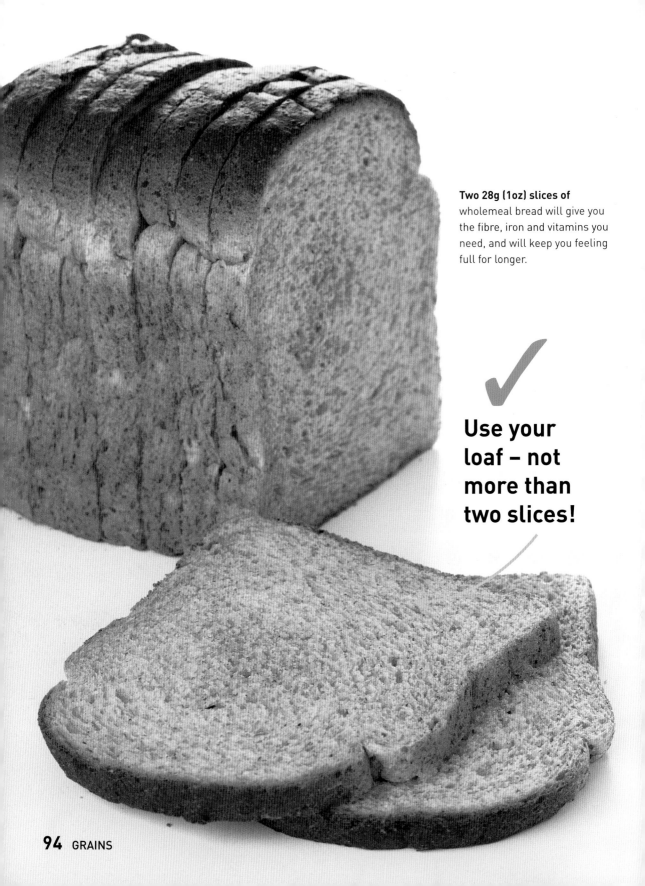

Two 28g (1oz) slices of wholemeal bread will give you the fibre, iron and vitamins you need, and will keep you feeling full for longer.

✓

Use your loaf – not more than two slices!

Bread

Does that delicious aroma coming from the supermarket bakery make your mouth water? Well, it's supposed to. Some supermarkets even make sure that the aroma is wafted through the entire store. Before you know it, there's a loaf in your trolley and you've already nibbled on it.

The bread basket arrives and, without thinking, you've eaten two rolls

Now picture this, you've had a long day and you're out to dinner with friends. The bread basket arrives. It's warm, inviting and, without thinking, you've eaten two rolls. We won't even mention the butter or oil you've had with it. What's wrong with this? The answer lies in the type of bread and the portion you eat.

White, brown, wholemeal and wholegrain are the most common types of bread but they're not the only ones. Add some variety to your life by choosing pitta bread for sandwiches or tortillas for wraps, enchiladas, burritos, fajitas and other Mexican foods. Baguettes are a traditional accompaniment for a French meal. Rye bread is a popular choice to eat with deli meats.

How much can I eat?

Plan on 28–57g (1–2oz) of bread a day. There are no British guidelines but the US government recommends we have three portions of whole grains a day. Aim to have at least half of your bread in the form of wholemeal or wholegrain to help you towards that recommended amount.

Choices to savour

There's plenty of choice when it comes to bread. Put the following at the top of your list: A 28g (1oz) slice of wholemeal or wholegrain bread has 69 calories, plus fibre, iron and vitamins • A 15cm (6in) wholemeal pitta bread will give you an acceptable 145 calories and some fibre • Flour

Nutritional analysis
per 57g (2oz) wholemeal bread portion as pictured

138 calories with 15 per cent from fat; **2.4g** fat, of which, **0.5g** saturated fat; **5.4g** protein; **0mg** cholesterol; **298mg** sodium; **3.8g** fibre

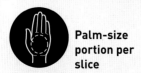

Palm-size portion per slice

tortillas are another option; a 15cm (6in) flour tortilla weighs in at 94 calories • A 28g (1oz) piece of baguette is 78 calories • A 28g (1oz) slice of rye bread is 73 calories

Choices to avoid

Plenty of perils await you in the bread basket. Watch out for these: White bread, especially with lots of butter. Skip the butter and spray with olive oil instead • Don't oversize that tortilla; a 25cm (10in) tortilla is 220 calories • Those anytime favourites – English muffins – are also to be avoided; just one is about 130 calories, and that's before you load it up with butter, jam or cream cheese

Watch the portion and get the fibre in the whole grain

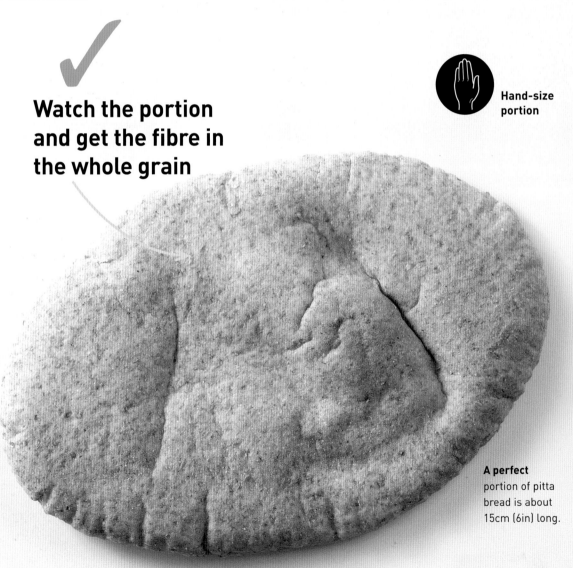

Hand-size portion

A perfect portion of pitta bread is about 15cm (6in) long.

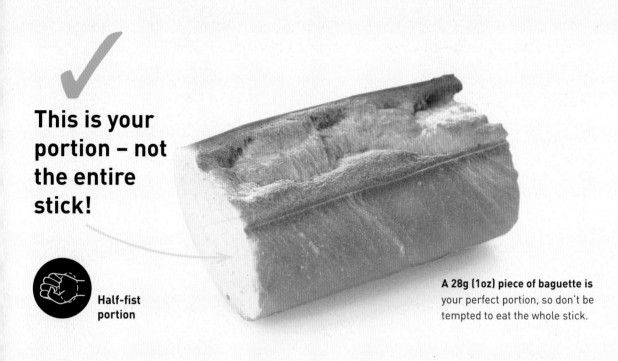

✓

This is your portion – not the entire stick!

Half-fist portion

A 28g (1oz) piece of baguette is your perfect portion, so don't be tempted to eat the whole stick.

Some vitamins and iron are added to refined grains, but essential fibre isn't

Healthy ways to enjoy

Read the labels. If a bread packet says 100 per cent wheat, this doesn't mean it's 100 per cent wholemeal. Most bread is made from wheat. The question is whether it's wholemeal (including the bran and germ) or refined. Refining gives a finer texture and longer shelf-life but also removes the dietary fibre, iron and many B vitamins. Many refined grains are enriched to compensate. For instance, certain B vitamins and iron are added back, but fibre, which is essential to our diet, isn't.

Take care that you're not fooled by the colour of the bread you're buying either. Some breads are brown because caramel colouring has been added.

The perils of garlic bread

Who doesn't enjoy their garlic bread? The problem is that garlic bread in many restaurants is a 227g (8oz) portion. It has about 810 calories with 38g of fat, usually saturated fat from butter and cheese. If you can't do without your garlic bread, eat it at home and make it yourself using 28g (1oz) of wholemeal baguette per portion. Spray the bread with olive oil spray and spread a crushed garlic clove over the slices. Toast until golden. That way you can enjoy your garlic bread and it will have only 185 calories and 4.5g fat.

Portion distortion: sandwiches

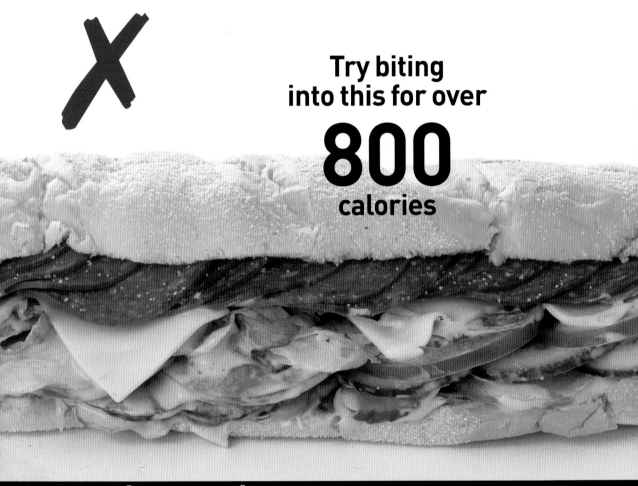

X

**Try biting
into this for over**

800

calories

oversize portion

Twenty years ago a toasted turkey sandwich was 320 calories. Today it's grown so much that it's more like 820 calories. That's 500 extra calories! Many sandwiches that you buy for lunch contain 227g (8oz) meat, which is the amount you should eat for two lunches. And, of course, the bread has grown in size to meet the meat, plus there's all that other stuff inside too – the heavy dose of melted cheese, for instance.

Tasty and filling yet only 363 calories

If your lunch-time sandwich has more than 113g (4oz) meat and two 28g (1oz) slices of bread, as pictured, save half for tomorrow.

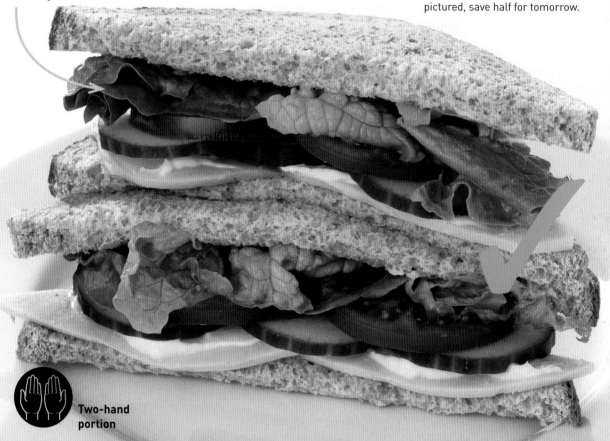

Two-hand portion

perfect portion

So what should you be eating? Order a sandwich made from just two 28g (1oz) slices of wholemeal bread and filled with a maximum of 113g (4oz) lean protein, such as lean meat or cooked fish. Then add in lettuce, tomatoes, cucumbers, drained roasted red peppers or other vegetables. Your lunch will be just as filling as before, but this time you'll be eating only around 363 calories and 8.1g fat.

Nutritional analysis
per turkey sandwich as pictured

363 calories with 20 per cent from fat; **8.1g** fat, of which, **1.4g** saturated fat; **39.9g** protein; **36.1** carbohydrate; **80mg** cholesterol; **465mg** sodium; **3.0g** fibre

Sandwich recipes

Sandwiches fit the bill for lunch. Choose two 28g (1oz) slices of wholemeal, rye or other wholegrain bread and sandwich them with one of your favourite fillings. These fillings are great for your Perfect Portion plan.

Grilled cheese (Serves 1)

This is a favourite with all ages. Just make it with two 28g (1oz) slices of wholemeal bread and 57g (2oz) reduced-fat Cheddar cheese.

Roast beef and horseradish (Serves 1)

Use 1 tbsp mayonnaise and 1 tbsp prepared horseradish with 113g (4oz) lean roast beef, turkey, chicken or lean ham on two 28g (1oz) slices of wholemeal bread.

Tuna fish (Serves 1)

Make your sandwich using 113g (4oz) tinned tuna packed in water and drained, tossed with 1 tbsp mayonnaise mixed with 1 tbsp lemon juice. Add 30g (1oz) grated celery, 40g (1½oz) chopped onion and 1 tbsp herbs. Serve on two 28g (1oz) slices of rye bread.

Egg salad (Serves 1)

For a healthy egg salad sandwich, mix 1 chopped hard-boiled egg, 2 chopped hard-boiled egg whites, 1 tbsp mayonnaise, 25g (¾oz) chopped celery and 1 tbsp chopped parsley. Spread it on two 28g (1oz) slices of wholegrain bread.

Roquefort cheese and walnut (Serves 1)

This sophisticated sandwich filling choice is fine as long as you're careful with the quantities. Mix 1 tbsp skimmed milk with 28g (1oz) Roquefort cheese. Spread between two 28g (1oz) slices of wholemeal bread and top with 1 tbsp chopped walnuts and ½ sliced apple.

Prawn salad sandwich (Serves 1)

Prawn salad is a favourite. Make by chopping 113g (4oz) bought cooked, peeled prawns with 31g (1oz) diced celery. Mix with 1 tbsp each mayonnaise and lime juice. Spread on two 28g (1oz) slices rye bread.

Sandwich your Portion Plan bread with one of these tasty fillings

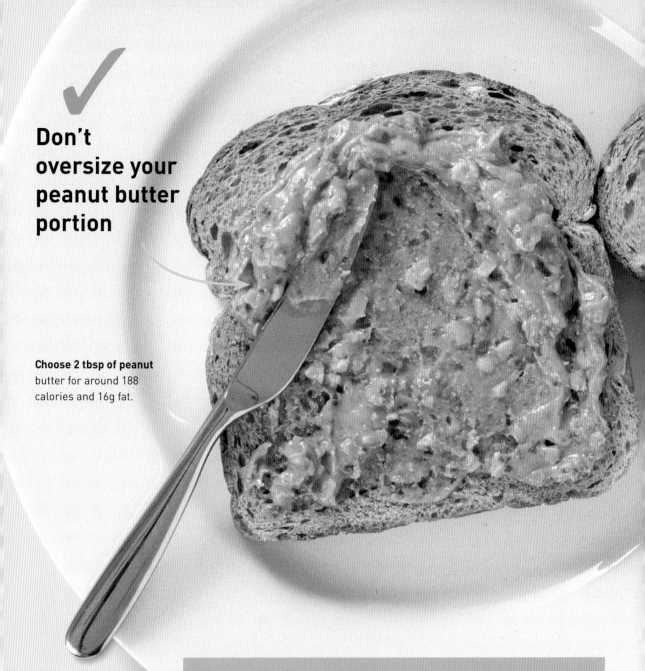

✓

Don't oversize your peanut butter portion

Choose 2 tbsp of peanut butter for around 188 calories and 16g fat.

Peanut butter

It turns out that the all-American PB and J (peanut butter and jam) sandwich is good for us as long as we don't oversize the portions. Stick to 2 tbsp peanut butter and 1 tbsp jam spread on two 28g (1oz) slices of wholemeal bread, and you'll be fine. That will give you a total of 382 calories and 18.4g of fat.

Portion distortion: tacos

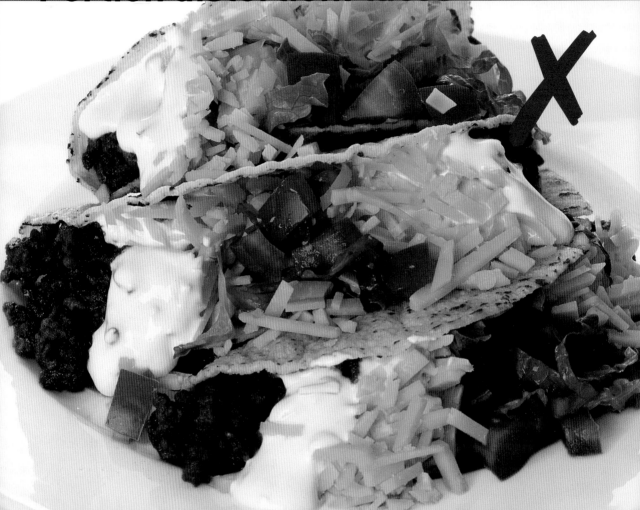

oversize portion

Those Tex-Mex tacos can really pile on the weight. And, who eats only one? A platter of three tacos with nachos and cheese can add up to over 1500 calories – and that's without the drink that goes with it. Just one 113g (4oz) taco like those pictured here also contains 350mg of sodium as well as 14g of fat, which is nearly a quarter what you should be having in a day. But, look opposite – you can have your taco and eat it.

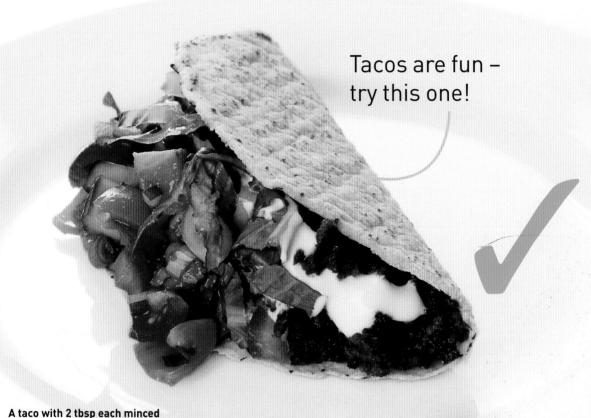

Tacos are fun –
try this one!

A taco with 2 tbsp each minced beef and salsa instead of cheese will cut your fat intake to around 10g and your sodium to 125mg.

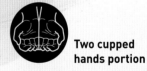

Two cupped hands portion

perfect portion

The trick with tacos is to watch your portions and order a taco containing salsa instead of Cheddar cheese. Yes, they do exist. Just eat one and you'll be cutting your fat intake down to less than 10g and your calories down to 220. Three are fine for a meal. Enjoy other Tex-Mex style foods but: order soft tortilla fajitas with grilled meat and vegetables; order burritos without rice and cheese.

Nutritional analysis
per taco portion as pictured

220 calories with 43 per cent from fat; **10.5g** fat, of which, **3.8g** saturated fat; **15.3g** protein; **41mg** cholesterol; **125mg** sodium; **1.1g** fibre

Breakfast pastries

Stop for a cup of coffee in the morning and you'll be faced with an enticing display of muffins, croissants and pastries. Hard to refuse, but look at what you're eating. The average 170g (6oz) muffin is about 500 calories as compared to 210 calories twenty years ago. Then a muffin used to be the size of an egg and would weigh 71g (2½oz). Even mini-muffins aren't that small today.

The same is true of buttery, flaky, melt-in-your-mouth croissants. These too have become oversized. A 99g (3½oz) buttery croissant is about 400 calories and 20g of fat (many of them saturated). It's like eating three slices (85g/3oz) of bread together with about five pats of butter.

And what about those doughnuts? They have expanded just like muffins and croissants. The average doughnut is twice the size it was two decades ago. Their size, plus the fact that they're filled with sugar and are deep-fried, make them a treat to enjoy just once in a while.

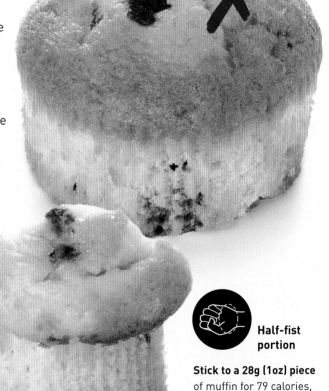

A 28g (1oz) bite will satisfy your muffin craving

Half-fist portion

Stick to a 28g (1oz) piece of muffin for 79 calories, 13.6g carbohydrates, 1.8g fat and 0.7g fibre.

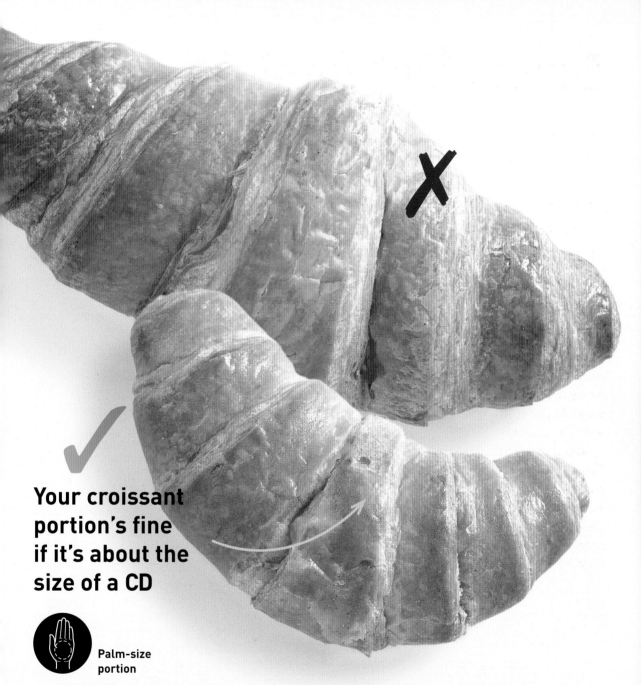

Your croissant portion's fine if it's about the size of a CD

Palm-size portion

Enjoy your croissant but keep it small: 28g (1oz) will give you 115 calories, 13g carbohydrates, 6g fat and 0.7g fibre.

Then there are those almond croissants and sugar, nut and fruit-laden Danish pastries. The average Danish, with 520 calories and 30g of fat, most of them saturated, will give you about the same amount of fat and calories as 237ml (8fl oz) of premium ice cream, while some almond croissants contain almost the same fat as an entire breakfast of two eggs, two slices of bacon and a slice of white, buttered toast. For instance, a 135g (4¾oz) almond croissant has 481 calories with 30.5g of fat.

The problem is that muffins, croissants and pastries aren't just on the breakfast or coffee-break menu. They're in airports, shopping centres, coffee and sandwich shops. And since they're bigger, we're bigger.

How much can I eat?

Whichever you choose, you should be aiming for about 28g (1oz). If you can't find a muffin that size, try half a mini muffin. When you buy a croissant, choose one that is about the size of a CD or cut a bigger one down to size. If you crave a doughnut, cut yourself a 28g (1oz) piece and freeze the rest or share it with some friends. The same is true of Danish pastries and almond croissants. If you must have a taste of Danish or of almond croissant, then make it just that – a taste. Cut yourself a 28g (1oz) piece and save the rest for later.

Choices to savour

Half a wholemeal English muffin is the best choice, with 67 calories. Add 1 tbsp reduced-fat cream cheese for an additional 35 calories or 28g (1oz) reduced-fat Cheddar cheese for 49 calories and a more nutritious choice.

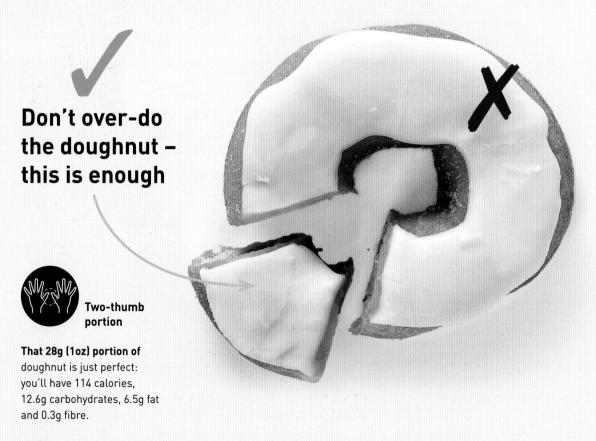

Don't over-do the doughnut – this is enough

Two-thumb portion

That 28g (1oz) portion of doughnut is just perfect: you'll have 114 calories, 12.6g carbohydrates, 6.5g fat and 0.3g fibre.

Or you can add 1 tbsp commercially prepared apple butter for 29 calories or 1 tbsp low-sugar apricot jam for 40 calories.

Choices to avoid

Jam- or cream-filled doughnuts • Flapjacks • Chocolate croissants • Sticky buns • Almond croissants • Super-sized muffins • Cheese or nut Danish pastries

Since breakfast pastries are bigger, we're bigger too

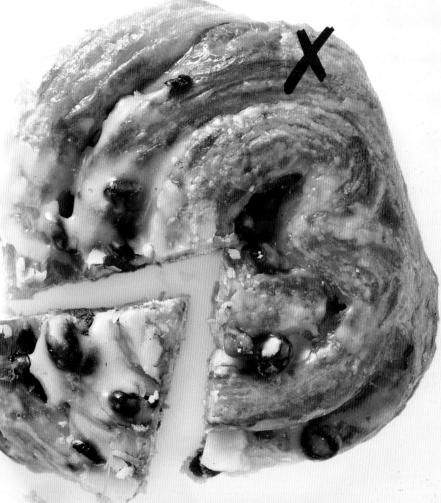

Perfect-portion a Danish – share it with a friend

Quarter-fist portion

Eat 28g (1oz) Danish now and save the rest for later. That way you'll have 105 calories, 13.6g carbohydrates, 5.2g fat and 0.5g fibre.

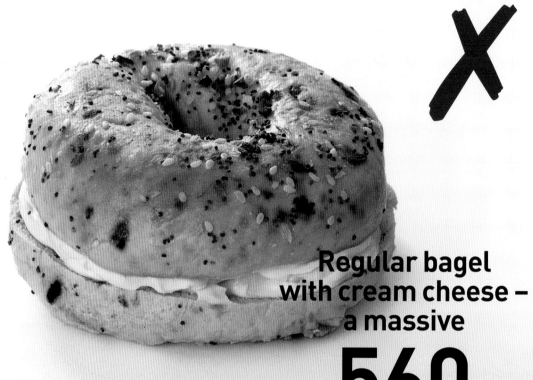

**Regular bagel
with cream cheese –
a massive**

560
calories!

oversize portion

Originally the size of a hockey puck, bagels now have the circumference of a CD. Eating just one is the same as eating five pieces of toast, which is enough portions of grain for the whole day. And as well as being bigger than they used to be, bagels are rarely eaten without a fat-filled topping. Choose an 11cm (4½in) bagel that weighs roughly 113g (4oz), add 57g (2oz) of cream cheese, and you'll be eating 560 calories.

Slim the bagel, slim the cheese

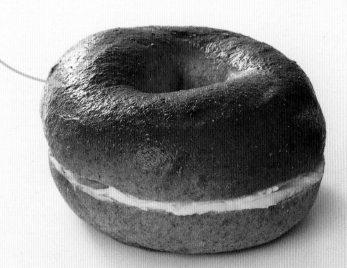

Reduced-fat cream cheese makes a 57g (2oz) bagel a healthy choice.

Palm-size portion

perfect portion

If you can't give up your bagel, choose a 7.5cm (3in) wholemeal bagel that weighs approximately 57g (2oz) and top it with 1 tbsp reduced-fat cream cheese to reach about 180 calories. If your bagel is larger, cut it in half and scoop out some of the inner bread. Or, only eat half. Alternatively, top with 28g (1oz) reduced-fat Cheddar, Emmenthal or other cheese, or with 1 tbsp fat-free yogurt.

Nutritional analysis
per 57g (2oz) bagel with cream cheese

178 calories with 19 per cent fat; **3.8g** fat, of which, **32.g** saturated fat; **6.4g** protein; **16mg** cholesterol; **318mg** sodium; **1.2g** fibre

Breakfast cereals

Breakfast in a hurry? Do you just pick up the cereal box and pour? And have you noticed that the bigger your bowl, the more you pour? And the more you pour the more you eat.... Well, the truth is you could be pouring 240g (8¾oz) of cereal and that could be as much as 800 calories, which is way above what you should be having.

Choosing 60g (2oz) low-fat granola and fat-free, low-sugar, flavoured yogurt will keep your fat and carbs intake under control.

This delicious breakfast is a great way to start your day

How much can I eat?

If you want to eat just the number of calories quoted on the cereal packet, then you need to forget about a big bowlful and cut your portion size down to about 30g (about 1oz).

Choices to savour

Look for a high-fibre cereal with at least 10g fibre per 30g (1oz). Bran cereals are the best choices • Look for whole grains. It's not just the fibre. Whole grains also supply nutrients and phytochemicals like magnesium, selenium, copper, manganese, vitamin E and phenolic acids that may protect against cancer, heart disease and diabetes • Hot cereals such as oatmeal are an excellent source of whole grains. The quality and quantity of the protein in oats is far superior to that of wheat and most other grains. But the most important nutritional advantage of oatmeal is the soluble fibre • Make your own delicious low-fat granola breakfast like the one pictured on the left (for the recipe, *see page 170*).

Choices to watch

Muesli or granola can be good choices, but watch the labels; many have a high sugar content • Look for low-fat muesli or granola with about 200 calories per 60g (2oz) and with 3g fat and 40g carbohydrates

Choices to avoid

Cereal's healthy image isn't true for many of the big-brand cereals because they contain high-fructose corn syrup and fat that replace protein and fibre. It's always important to read the labels and see exactly how healthy your cereal is.

Healthy ways to enjoy

• Don't spoil a good breakfast cereal choice with lots of extra sugar. Instead add sweetness with a few raisins, apricots or other dried fruits.
• You can also add 53–83g (1¾–3oz) fresh fruit such as blueberries, pomegranate seeds, strawberries, pears and apples.
• Cinnamon adds sweetness without sugar.

> The truth is you could be pouring as many as 800 calories into your cereal bowl

Nutritional analysis

per 60g (2oz) granola cereal, yogurt and almonds as pictured

415 calories with 20 per cent from fat; **9.3g** fat, of which, **1.4g** saturated fat; **21.1g** protein; **5mg** cholesterol; **324mg** sodium; **4.8g** fibre

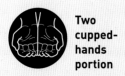

Two cupped-hands portion

Grain meal accompaniments

Make 157g (5¾oz) quinoa your choice and have 190 calories and 35g carbohydrates.

Three-quarter fist portion

A 182g (6½oz) portion of tasty bulgur wheat will give you 151 calories and 37.8g carbohydrates.

Fist-size portion

Savour your grains – but in moderation

A 146g (5¼oz) portion of healthy wholegrain brown rice is 162 calories and 33.6g carbohydrates.

Three-quarter fist portion

Love that rich paella or creamy risotto? Do you enjoy trying other grain meal accompaniments such as buckwheat or bulgur wheat? Without thinking about it we can pile these on our plates and break our portion bank, sometimes eating close to 1000 calories at one meal. How far do you think you have to run to work all that off? There's no need to give up these foods. Just eyeball the photo and follow the recommendations here to enjoy perfect portions.

Enjoy a perfect portion of 119g (4¼oz) white rice for 154 calories and 33.4g carbohydrates.

Three-quarter fist portion

How much can I eat?

The portions vary according to the type of grain you're eating: White rice 119g (4¼oz) cooked • Brown rice 146g (5¼oz) cooked • Wild rice 123g (4½oz) cooked • Bulgur wheat 182g (6½oz) cooked • Buckwheat 126g (4½oz) cooked • Quinoa 157g (5¾oz) cooked

Choices to savour

Brown rice • Wild rice • Bulgur wheat • Buckwheat • Quinoa

Choices to watch

White rice • Jasmine (Thai) rice • Polenta • Couscous • Basmati rice

Choices to avoid

A plateful of fried rice or risotto

Healthy ways to enjoy

- Brown rice versus white, which should we eat? Both types are nutritious, low in sodium and high in potassium, which regulates the body's water balance. But brown rice is a wholegrain rice that's been milled so the bran stays intact, which means that it's healthier. It contains 18 per cent of the daily protein requirement and triple the fibre of white rice. White rice has been processed so the bran layers and embryo have been stripped off. And it's often polished, too, which removes the healthy dust that results from the stripping process.
- Brown rice takes about 45 minutes to cook, but you can still enjoy the health benefits of brown rice by selecting 10- or 30-minute brown rice. This rice has been par-cooked to save you some preparation time.
- Bulgur and quinoa are ancient, nutrient-packed grains. Soak bulgur in water, drain and serve with a salad dressing; or cook for 15 minutes in water, then dress. Quinoa has a nutty flavour and cooks like rice.

Pasta

Serve an entire plate of pasta to an Italian as his main course and he'll wonder why. In Italy, pasta is served as a side dish or first course in amounts of about 105g (3¾oz) cooked. Portions in other countries like the UK have grown so big they cover a large plate and they're served as the main dish, usually with a tomato sauce and cheese.

Order a main course of pasta and you may be eating as much as 700 calories for that dish alone. Together with the rest of the meal, this could put you at over 1200 calories, or nearly a day's worth of calories. What's more, if you eat a dish such as Fettuccine Alfredo, which has butter, Parmesan cheese and cream added to the pasta, you'll be eating as much saturated fat as there is in about 473ml (16½fl oz) of ice cream.

How much can I eat?
Stick to 170g (6oz) cooked pasta, and go easy on the sauce and cheese.

Choices to savour
Whole-wheat pasta such as spaghetti, fettuccine, penne, egg noodles, angel hair, lasagne, shells, elbows and spirals • Eat with marinara sauce, tomato-based pasta or pizza sauces

Choices to avoid
Pasta dishes loaded with butter and cream such as: Fettuccine Alfredo • Spaghetti Carbonara • Lasagne • Pasta with more than 25g (¾oz) Parmesan on top • Pasta with fat-laden ragú (meat) sauce • Cannelloni

Test yourself
Try measuring your normal portion of pasta. You may find that your serving equals three to four times the recommended portion.

Healthy ways to enjoy
Whole-wheat pasta is slowly digested and is full of good nutrients, many of which have been removed from white-flour pasta. It's also more filling than white-flour pasta and so helps to curb your appetite.

Aim to eat your pasta as a side dish with other vegetables

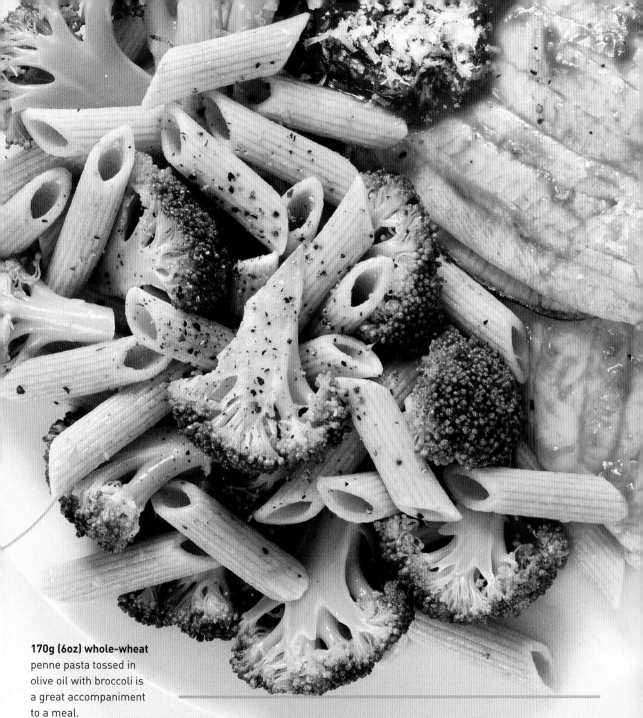

170g (6oz) whole-wheat penne pasta tossed in olive oil with broccoli is a great accompaniment to a meal.

Two cupped-hands portion

Nutritional analysis
per 170g (6oz) whole-wheat pasta with broccoli portion as pictured

379 calories, with 39 per cent from fat; of which, **3g** saturated fat; **14.4g** protein; **49.9g** carbohydrate; **4mg** cholesterol; **134mg** sodium; **3.9g** fibre (*see page 176 for nutritional analysis of whole plate*)

Portion distortion: pizza

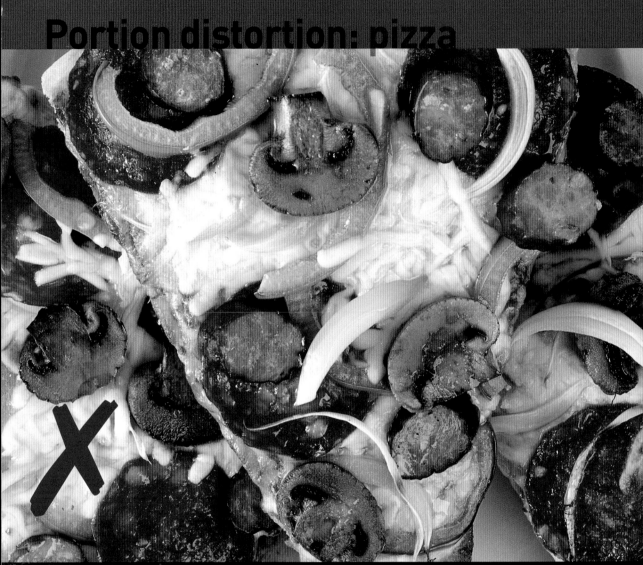

X

oversize portion

Have a bottle of beer and four slices of a 36cm (14in) pizza with double cheese and sausage – the life-size pizza's pictured here but we couldn't fit it all on the page! – and you'll be getting 2100 calories. That's 50 per cent more than an entire day's calorie allowance. Even a two-slice lunch special with a cola can add up to 1000 calories. Whichever you choose, today's fast-food pizza can be a calorie disaster.

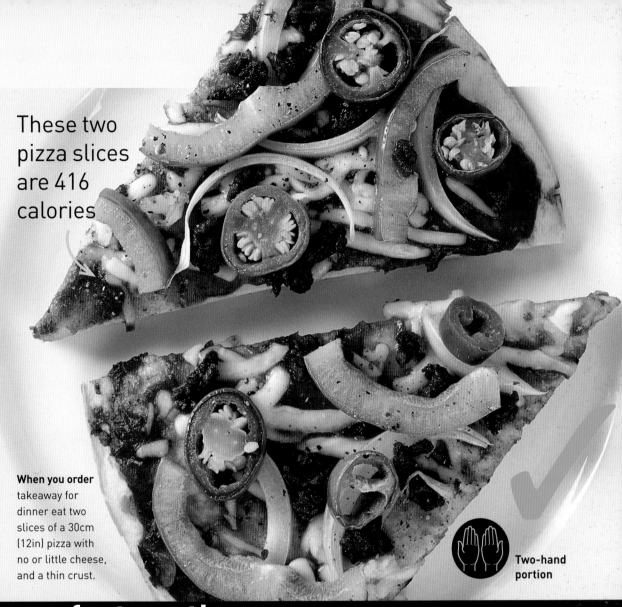

These two pizza slices are 416 calories

When you order takeaway for dinner eat two slices of a 30cm (12in) pizza with no or little cheese, and a thin crust.

Two-hand portion

perfect portion

Crave pizza? It's healthier to make your own. Sauté 85g (3oz) sliced low-fat turkey sausages for 2 minutes in a non-stick frying pan. Spoon 125g (4½oz) low-sodium pizza sauce over a 15cm (6in) pizza base, then add the sausage, plus 18g (¾oz) sliced mushrooms, 23g (¾oz) sliced green pepper, and 29g (1oz) sliced onion. Place on a foil-lined baking tray, sprinkle with 2 tbsp reduced-fat mozzarella, and grill for 4 minutes.

Nutritional analysis
per two-slice pizza portion as pictured

416 calories with 20 per cent from fat; **9.2g** fat, of which, **2.5g** saturated fat; **20.5g** protein; **23mg** cholesterol; **622mg** sodium; **4.7g** fibre

sweet treats

What's dinner without dessert, a summer's day out without an ice cream or a cup of coffee without a piece of cake? Most desserts, sweets and chocolate have lots of sugar and little nutritional value. With Perfect Portion you can eat a little of what you crave – chocolate cake, apple pie, brownies, cookies and even chocolate. Just a taste ends your meal on a sweet note and you won't need to feel deprived. More than that adds lots of empty calories with little nutritional value. To discover how to incorporate the occasional sweet treat in your perfect portion plan on a regular basis, see my Seven-Day Eating Plan on pages 160–180.

Cake and desserts

Deep down we all suspect that we should stop eating dessert and this is why. A 15cm (6in) high serving of frosted carrot cake or chocolate fudge cake at a restaurant can weigh in at 1500 calories. A slice of plain or fruit-glazed cheesecake can be 710 calories.

Unless you're one of the lucky few who don't have a sweet tooth, we all find it really, really difficult to give up desserts. And the problem for most of us is that denying ourselves dessert usually has the effect of making us want more. So what are we to do? The answer is don't give up dessert but know the right portion to have. Everyone loves a little sweet at the end of a meal, but keep it small.

We all find it really, really difficult to give up desserts

How much can I eat?
Think in terms of slicing your cake no wider than two fingers and if you are in a restaurant, cut that much from the serving and share the rest or take it home to eat with the family the next day.

Choices to savour
Bread pudding 57g (2oz) • Carrot cake (frosted) 28g (1oz) • Chocolate cake 28g (1oz) • Chocolate cheesecake 28g (1oz) • Fruit cheesecake 28g (1oz) • Plain cheesecake 28g (1oz) • Flan (Crème caramel) 57g (2oz) • Fruit sorbet 88g (3¼oz) • Peach cobbler 57g (2oz) • Pecan pie 2.5cm (1in) slice weighing 28g (1oz) • Tiramisu 57g (2oz)

Choices to avoid
Large portions of any desserts. Use the choices to savour as a guide.

Healthy ways to enjoy
If you really can't do without dessert, some choices are healthier than others. Tempted by a piece of strawberry shortcake? Satisfy your sweet tooth with a bowl of fresh strawberries, either on their own or with 1 tbsp whipped cream. Do you hanker for a calorific peach cobbler? Eat a dish of sliced fresh peaches served with plain fat-free yogurt instead. Another sweet way to end a meal without adding a lot of calories is to order a herbal tea or flavoured coffee and add skimmed milk.

This portion of frosted carrot cake only contains 103 calories for 28g (1oz).

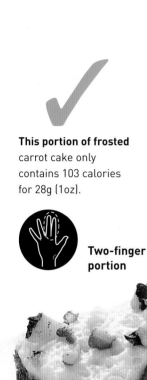

Two-finger portion

A taster of chocolate fudge cake is allowed and contains 103 calories for 28g (1oz).

Two-finger portion

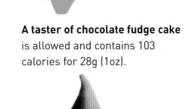

Choose strawberry cheesecake in a portion with only 108 calories for 28g (1oz).

Two-finger portion

Apple pie

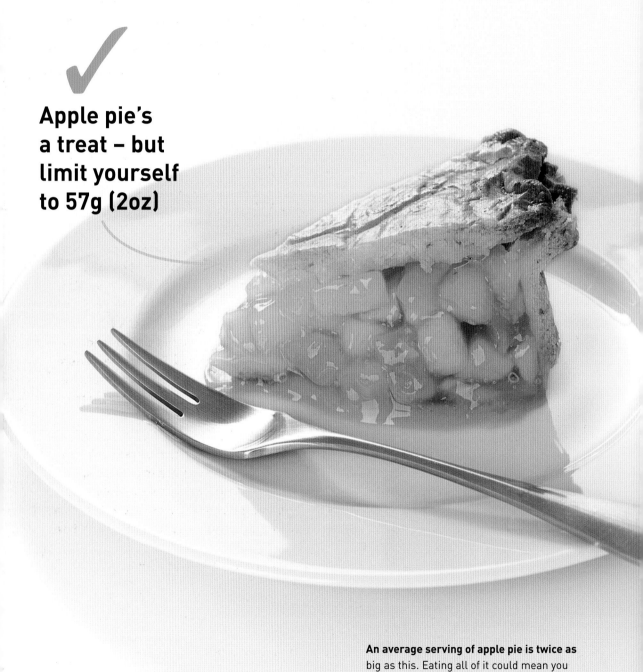

Apple pie's
a treat – but
limit yourself
to 57g (2oz)

An average serving of apple pie is twice as big as this. Eating all of it could mean you have to run for half an hour to burn off the nearly 300 calories it contains.

Eating apple pie isn't necessarily the best way to get more fruit into your diet

Are you choosing apple pie as dessert thinking that you are making a healthy choice? We all know we should be getting more fruit into our diets, but apple pie isn't necessarily the best way to do it, especially if your portion size is way above what it should be. Eat an average 113g (4oz) serving of apple pie and you could be helping yourself to 14g of fat and 332mg of sodium as well as nearly 300 calories.

How much can I eat?
Whichever type of fruit pie you opt for – apple, cherry, peach, blackberry or rhubarb – limit yourself to a 57g (2oz) slice, which is about the width of three fingers or the amount that would fit into a cupped hand.

Healthy ways to enjoy
If you want your apple pie but would like a healthier option, make your own with a granola crust, fresh apples, and a low-sugar glaze. The granola crust is not only healthier than a regular pastry crust, but also has a much lower carb count.

Spray an 18–20cm (7–8in) pie plate with olive oil spray. Place 60g (2oz) low-fat granola, 42g (1½oz) digestive biscuit crumbs and 3 tbsp rapeseed oil in the bowl of a food processor. Process the mixture until the oil is mixed into the dry ingredients to form crumbs. Press the crumbs into the base of the pie plate. Refrigerate while preparing the other ingredients.

Meanwhile, preheat the oven to 190°C (375°F/Gas 5). Peel, core, quarter and slice 908g (2lb) tart cooking apples and use them to fill the pie plate. Mix 2 tbsp brown sugar and 1 tsp cinnamon together and sprinkle on top of the apples. Bake for 45 minutes until the apples are cooked through. Heat 6 tbsp reduced-sugar apricot jam and 2 tbsp water together in a small pan to form a glaze, then spread over the cooked pie. Serve hot or cold.

This recipe makes 10 servings at 150 calories per serving.

Nutritional analysis
per 57g (2oz) apple pie portion as pictured

134 calories with 42 per cent from fat, of which, **2.2g** saturated fat; **1.1g** protein; **19.3g** carbohydrate; **0mg** cholesterol; **151mg** sodium; **0.9g** fibre

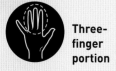
Three-finger portion

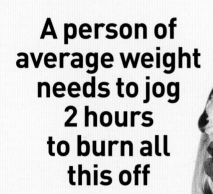

A person of average weight needs to jog 2 hours to burn all this off

oversize portion

Throughout the world ice cream is a favourite dessert or snack. Have your ice cream, but watch the size and the extras. Eat a three-scoop serving of pecan and toffee ice cream topped with 2 tbsp chocolate fudge sauce, 2 tbsp walnuts, 60g (2oz) sweetened whipped cream and a cherry on top, and you've reached a whopping 1400 calories. That's an entire day's worth of calories.

Can't resist an ice cream but don't want to jog for two hours? Then make sure you choose the perfect portion. An average 68g (2½oz) portion of light, no-sugar-added ice cream – or about one ice-cream scoop in a cone – will only give you 145 calories.

Perfect-portion your ice cream to just 145 calories

Nutritional analysis
per 68g (2½oz) ice cream portion in cone

145 calories with 34 per cent from fat; **5.5g** fat, of which, **2.8g** saturated fat; **3.5g** protein; **18mg** cholesterol; **97mg** sodium; **0.7g** fibre

Half-fist portion

Eat 68g (2½oz) light ice cream in a cone and you can jog off those calories in around ten minutes.

Brownies and cookies

The all-American brownie is a universal favourite. The original 20cm (8in) square brownie tin made sixteen brownies. But order a brownie at a restaurant today and you are likely to get a 10cm (4in) brownie that's the equivalent of about 550 calories. And if it's made with 1 tbsp nuts, it will reach 600 calories. Add a scoop of vanilla ice cream on top, and it brings you up to 850 calories.

There's the same problem with cookies, too. How many do you eat at one sitting? Two of today's 'average' cookies will set you back 525 calories – or enough calories for a meal. And that's for an average cookie. Many cookies nowadays are oversized to about 13cm (5in) in diameter. That gives you about 300 calories plus – for just one cookie.

How much can I eat?
Enjoy your brownie but plan on just a 2.5cm (1in) square. This 28g (1oz) piece will have about 115 calories.

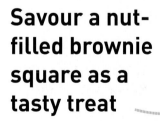

Savour a nut-filled brownie square as a tasty treat

Have only 115 calories and 4.7g of fat when you eat this 2.5cm (1in) 28g (1oz) square of brownie with nuts.

Two-thumb portion

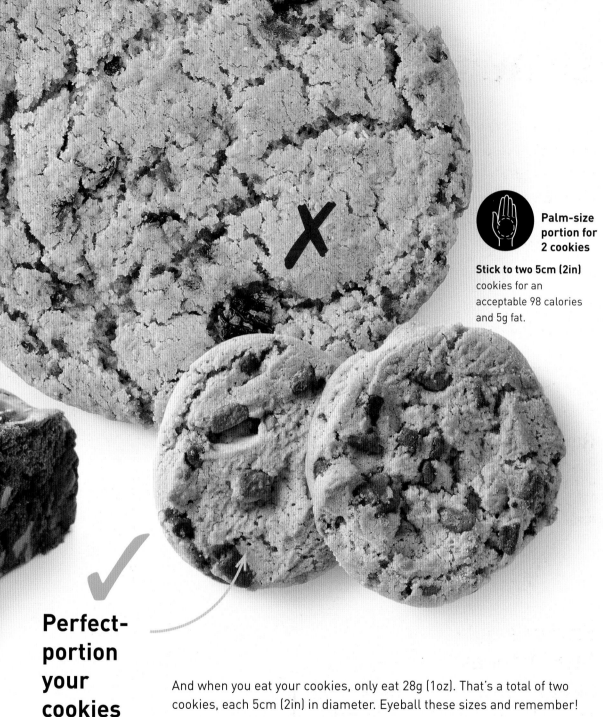

Palm-size portion for 2 cookies

Stick to two 5cm (2in) cookies for an acceptable 98 calories and 5g fat.

Perfect-portion your cookies

And when you eat your cookies, only eat 28g (1oz). That's a total of two cookies, each 5cm (2in) in diameter. Eyeball these sizes and remember!

Healthy ways to enjoy

Choose wholegrain cookies. They may have the same calories as regular cookies, but they are healthier for you because they are made with wholegrain flour (*see Healthy ways to enjoy, page 97*).

Chocolate and sweets

Chocoholics rejoice. The ancient Mayans used to refer to chocolate as the food of the gods. Today, research has shown that they may have been right. Chocolate has some beneficial health effects and is not necessarily a food taboo. Chocolate makes a holiday festive and nowadays, dark chocolate is even considered good for you.

Sweets are a different matter though. They are made mostly from sugar. This means they have lots of calories but few nutrients, which is why they are considered 'empty' calories.

How much can I eat?

So, how much chocolate and sweets can you eat? About 100 calories of dark chocolate (not milk). That's 28g (1oz). But don't make eating sweets a habit. Think in terms of one small sweet on occasion. If your sweet tooth is calling for sweets, try a piece of fruit.

Choices to savour

Dark chocolate (minimum 70 per cent cocoa solids) • Low-calorie sweets • Sugar-free sweets

Choices to avoid

Milk chocolate • White chocolate

Healthy ways to enjoy

- If you really can't give up your chocolate, choose dark chocolate over milk or white. Why? Dark chocolate contains far more of the antioxidants that help protect against heart disease and high blood pressure. In fact, it contains twice the amount that are in milk chocolate. So why not have white chocolate? Because it's a less healthy choice. It contains more carbohydrates – mostly in the form of sugar – and has less protein than other types of chocolate.
- Another way to satisfy your yearning for chocolate is to combine it with fruit. Why not try strawberries and fresh orange segments dipped in melted dark chocolate, for example?

Dark chocolate contains disease-fighting antioxidants

Yes! You can even enjoy the occasional chocolate moment

If you eat this entire chocolate bar, as well as nearly 30g sugar, you'll be having 551 calories and 41.1g fat, of which, 24.2g are saturated.

Savour the taste of a 28g (1oz) guilt-free piece of dark chocolate from time to time.

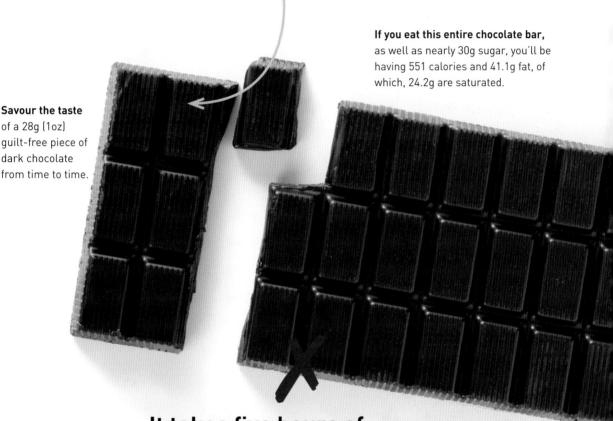

It takes five hours of high-impact aerobics to burn all these calories

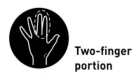

Two-finger portion

Nutritional analysis
per 28g (1oz) dark chocolate portion as pictured

145 calories with 70 per cent from fat; **11.2g** fat, of which, **6.6g** saturated fat; **1.3g** protein; **0mg** cholesterol; **0mg** sodium; **2g** fibre

drinks and snacks

How many calories a day do you drink? We're advised to drink 1.8 litres (64fl oz) of water a day – that's eight 237ml (8fl oz) glasses. But, can we count coffee, tea and soft drinks? If so, how many calories will that add? While water is a great choice, herbal teas, calorie-free, flavoured water and sparkling water are also good. Tea is thought to have beneficial properties. But what about alcohol? In moderation, it can be good for us. And then there are your snacks. Have you added up the calories you nibble on while you're having a drink, when you're having a snack at the cinema or while you're watching TV? Read the following pages and you'll find that we have some tips for you. All the answers and your perfect portions are here.

Non-alcohol drinks

We know that we should drink 1.8 litres (64fl oz) of liquid a day. The question is what can we drink that won't add calories and sugar to our menu? Reaching for water when thirsty is the best answer, but sometimes you simply hanker for a drink with more flavour.

Choices to savour

The following choices are calorie-free or almost calorie-free: Water • Sparkling water • Flavoured (no-calorie) water • Herbal teas • Green, black and red tea • One 237ml (8fl oz) cup of coffee with sugar substitute and no milk is 5 calories

Choices to watch

Some of these choices are deceptive: Tea or coffee with milk and sugar – the milk and sugar add calories • Bottled instant iced tea made with sugar can have 90 calories for a 237ml (8fl oz) glass • Some 237ml (8fl oz) chai drinks can have 150 calories • Diet drinks have almost no calories but very high concentrates of sugar substitutes – drink one a day at most • A 355ml (12fl oz) sparkling, sugary soft drink can add about 150 calories to your daily diet • Apple juice, orange juice, pineapple juice and grape juice are favourite fruit drinks – a 177ml (6fl oz) glass will add about 100 calories to your day (*see page 91*)

Choices to avoid

A giant 710ml (24fl oz) portion of regular cola will give you 292 calories • A 570ml (20fl oz) whole milk latte adds up to 350 calories • Watch those frappes and other speciality coffee drinks with whipped cream – a 710ml (24fl oz) speciality frappe can add about 700 calories to your day

What can we drink that won't add calories and sugar?

Nutritional analysis
per 237ml (8fl oz) diet cola portion

0 calories with 0 per cent from fat; **0g** fat, of which, **0g** saturated fat; **0g** protein; **0mg** cholesterol; **26mg** sodium; **0g** fibre

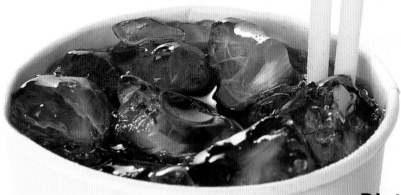

Diet cola contains no calories – but only have one a day

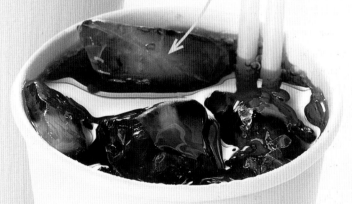

Choose a 237ml (8fl oz) diet cola over regular cola in any size. There is some evidence that cola may leach calcium from our bones, so stick to one perfect portion a day.

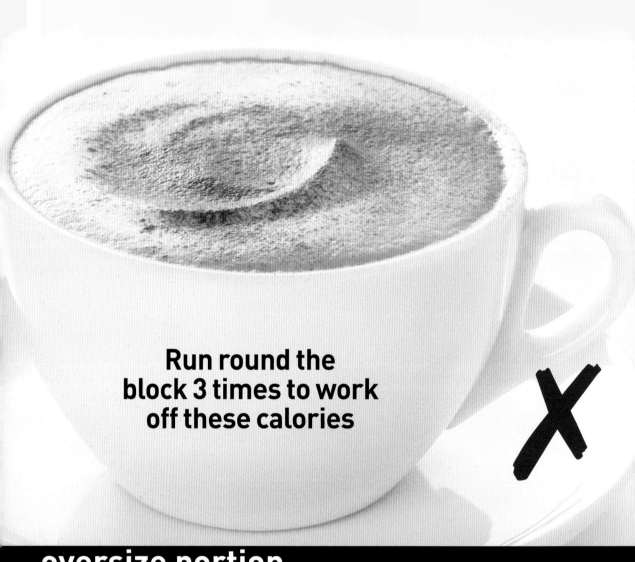

**Run round the
block 3 times to work
off these calories**

oversize portion

Would you believe that even your favourite morning coffee has been growing to unhealthy proportions? Your parents enjoyed a 230ml (8fl oz) cup of coffee with whole milk. Even adding a teaspoon of sugar, that totalled only 45 calories. Today we don't think twice about buying a giant 570ml (20fl oz) latte with chocolate powder sprinkled on top. That will give you a massive 340 calories – and it's only a drink!

Relax on the sofa with your perfect portion coffee

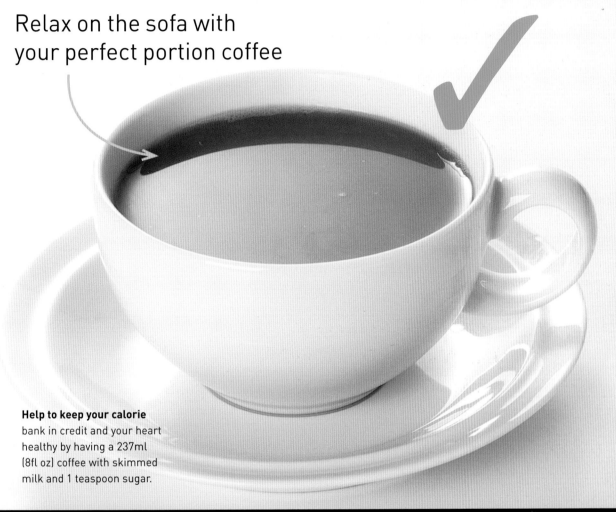

Help to keep your calorie bank in credit and your heart healthy by having a 237ml (8fl oz) coffee with skimmed milk and 1 teaspoon sugar.

perfect portion

Wouldn't you far sooner be doing something other than running round the block in your lunch break? If your answer is 'yes', then choose a 237ml (8fl oz) cup of coffee made with skimmed milk and wean yourself to 1 level tsp of sugar. That way your calorie intake will drop to a healthy 32 calories. But even this perfect portion needs to be watched. Too much coffee with caffeine can be harmful.

Nutritional analysis
per 237ml (8fl oz) coffee as pictured

32 calories with 2 per cent from fat; **0.1g** fat, of which, **0g** saturated fat; **1.3g** protein; **1mg** cholesterol; **21mg** sodium; **0g** fibre

Alcoholic drinks

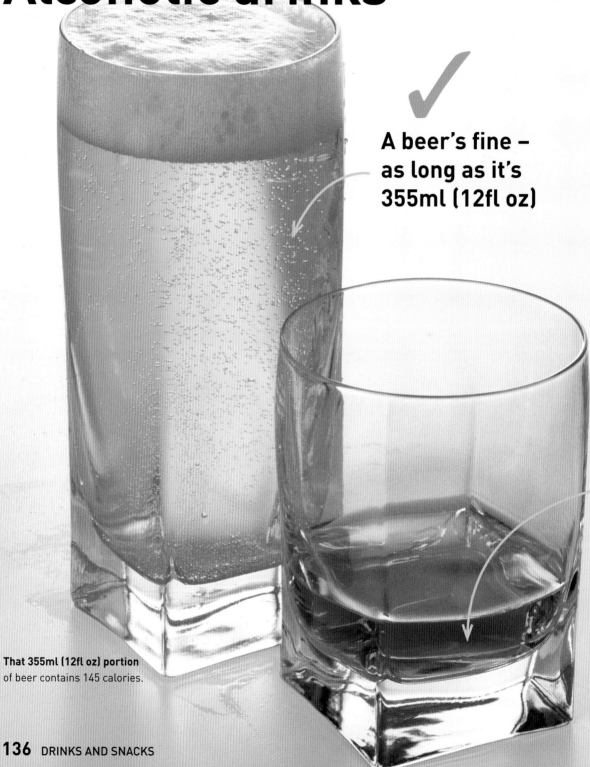

A beer's fine – as long as it's 355ml (12fl oz)

That 355ml (12fl oz) portion of beer contains 145 calories.

The debate about alcohol has been going on for centuries. Is it good for you or bad? The answer lies in the quantity you consume. Some research reveals that moderate drinking is good for the heart and circulatory system, while heavy drinking is a major cause of preventable deaths as it can damage the liver and heart.

Avoid the many 'empty calories' that alcohol contains

Remember when drinking alcohol, it doesn't make you feel full. It contains what's known as 'empty' calories. It can increase your appetite, too, which is why an alcoholic drink is also called an aperitif.

How much can I have?

From the health point of view, you should always follow government guidelines and stick to drinking moderate amounts. The Department of Health advises men to drink no more than 3–4 units a day, and women no more than 2–3 units a day. As examples of units, a 177ml (6fl oz) glass of wine is 2 units; a 570ml (20fl oz) glass of bitter is 3 units.

Choices to savour

These choices keep you within the government recommendations and won't break the calorie bank: A 148ml (5fl oz) glass of red or white wine averages 125 calories • A 355ml (12fl oz) beer has about 145 calories • A 355ml (12fl oz) light beer has about 100 calories • Most spirits – such as vodka, whisky, scotch, gin, and so on – are about 90–100 calories per 30ml (1fl oz)

Choices to avoid

Once you add flavourings to your spirits, you add calories, too: Add 355ml (12fl oz) tonic to a 44ml jigger (1½fl oz) of gin or 355ml (12fl oz) cola to a 44ml jigger (1½fl oz) of rum and you're drinking about 230–250 calories • A martini cocktail will set you back about 375 calories • Frozen daiquiris are tasty, but watch the amount of sugary mixture that goes into them – it can be as much as 227 calories for 118ml (4fl oz) • Tex-Mex margaritas and Caribbean mojitos are popular drinks, but a margarita is about 350 calories for 237ml (8fl oz) and a mojito can be 205 calories for 118ml (4fl oz) • Piña coladas made with coconut cream can pack on the calories – about 526 of them for 207ml (7fl oz) • The same goes for a rum punch, a favourite to have while sitting on the beach. It is usually made with sugary fruit juices and can pack 447 calories for 355ml (12fl oz)

Your healthy choice is just a finger of whisky

Whisky lovers take care. Stick to 44ml (1½fl oz) for 105 calories.

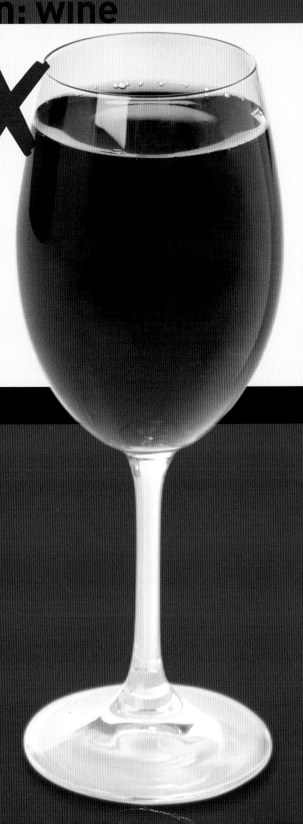

Portion distortion: wine

Have you noticed how that 'innocent' glass of wine has grown?

oversize portion

Order a glass of your favourite wine with dinner and prepare for a shock. Wine glasses are much bigger than they used to be and you'll drink the entire glassful. And maybe order a second glass, too. But how many calories will you be having? Drink the 237ml (8fl oz) glass shown on this page and that will be a hefty 168 calories. Some places even serve wine in a 355ml (12fl oz) glass containing 252 calories.

Stick to just one 148ml (5fl oz) portion

perfect portion

The way forward is to buck the trend and order a 148ml (5fl oz) glass – and don't order a second one. That way you'll be cutting down your calorie intake to 106 calories and you can enjoy your main course guilt-free. Other ways to enjoy your wine are: have a wine spritzer – a longer drink – made with sparkling water and wine; if you are going to a long cocktail party, start with sparkling water with a twist of lemon or lime, or with a diet drink.

That 148ml (5fl oz) wine portion doesn't only hold your calories in check; it keeps your drinking within the moderate recommended levels, too.

Nutritional analysis
per 148ml (5fl oz) glass red wine as pictured

106 calories with 0 per cent from fat; **0.3g** protein; **2.5g** carbohydrate; **1.4mg** sodium

Snacks and nibbles

It's so easy to buy a bag of crisps or tortilla chips and dip into them while you're watching TV, having a drink or at the pictures. Before you know it, the whole bag has gone. This kind of snack can seriously damage your daily calorie total and will add some unhealthy fats to your diet, too.

Watch what you take when you dip into those snacks

How much can I eat?

Generally speaking, you can enjoy your snacks as long as you limit your portion to 28g (1oz).

Choices to savour

The protein and monounsaturated fat in nuts make them a better snack alternative than crisps. Try these when you feel a snack urge coming on: Dry-roasted peanuts have 170 calories per 28g (1oz) – that's about 40 peanuts • Almonds have 163 calories per 28g (1oz) – or 23 whole pieces • Pecans have 196 calories per 28g (1oz) – about 20 halves • Walnuts have 185 calories per 28g (1oz) – or 14 halves • Pretzels have 108 calories per 28g (1oz)

Choose a 28g (1oz) portion of dry-roasted peanuts for 170 calories and 14g fat.

Cupped-hand portion

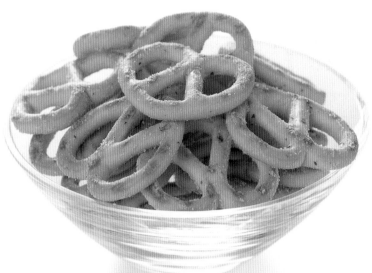

This 28g (1oz) portion of pretzels will give you 108 calories and 0.8g fat.

Cupped-hand portion

Choices to avoid

Watch your portions with these: Crisps: that 113g (4oz) bag at lunch can add about 600 calories to the meal, but a 28g (1oz) portion has only around 150 calories • A 227g (8oz) bag of tortilla chips contains about 1100 calories, so eat only 28g (1oz) to come in under 140 calories

Healthy ways to enjoy

As well as limiting your snack portions, don't forget about vegetables as a snack. You can buy most of them ready-to-eat from the supermarket. Try carrot and celery sticks, broccoli and cauliflower florets, sliced peppers, or edamame (soya beans). And then there's also the option of having around fifteen olives as a snack.

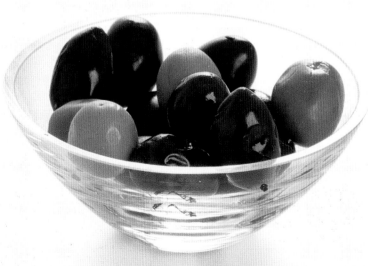

A portion of fifteen olives contains 75 calories and 7.1g fat.

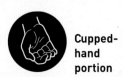
Cupped-hand portion

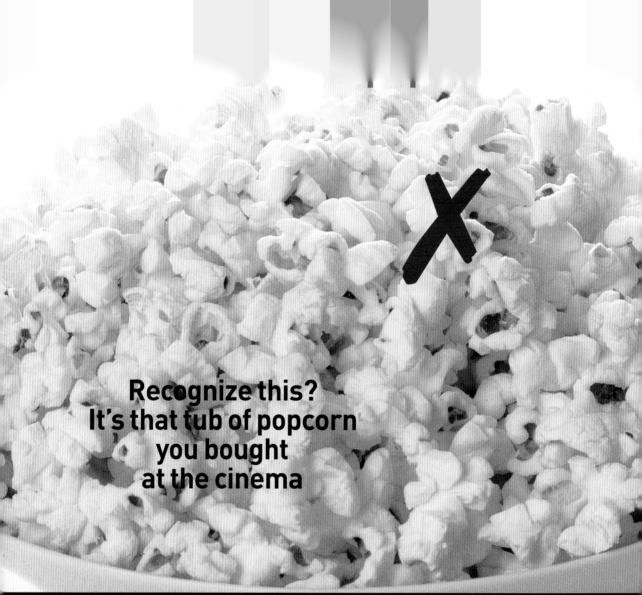

Recognize this?
It's that tub of popcorn
you bought
at the cinema

oversize portion

Go into a cinema today and the smell of popcorn draws you right to the refreshments kiosk. Twenty years ago a box of popcorn was about 55g (2oz) and 275 calories. Today a tub of popcorn can be as big as 132g (4¾oz) and can have as many as 660 calories – and that doesn't count the free refills. Order buttered popcorn and you could be adding another 200 calories to your film night out.

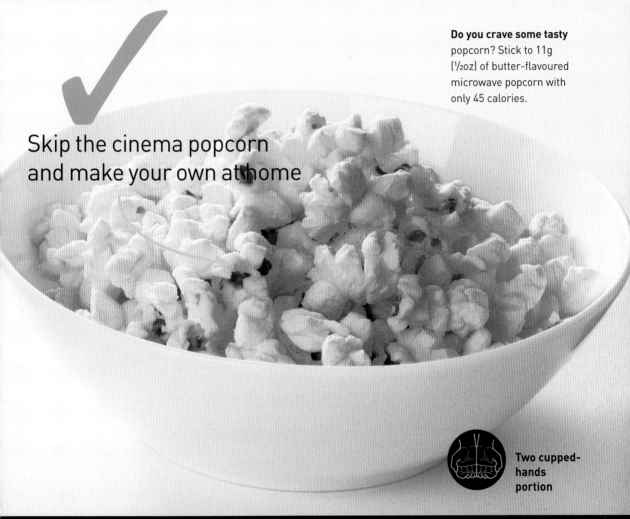

Skip the cinema popcorn
and make your own at home

Do you crave some tasty popcorn? Stick to 11g (½oz) of butter-flavoured microwave popcorn with only 45 calories.

Two cupped-hands portion

perfect portion

In contrast, butter-flavoured microwave popcorn contains roughly 45 calories for 11g (½oz) or about the same calories as the equivalent weight of popcorn of twenty years ago. To make a healthy eating choice, plan on 22–33g (¾–1oz) of popcorn popped in vegetable oil. Make sure it has not been popped in oil containing trans fats. Better still, try and opt for air-popped popcorn.

Nutritional analysis
per 11g (½oz) popcorn portion as pictured

55 calories with 51 per cent from fat; of which, **0.5g** saturated fat; **1g** protein; **6.3g** carbohydrates; **0mg** cholesterol; **97mg** sodium; **1.1g** fibre

Dip recipes

Dips make great snacks – and are easy to serve when friends stop by or at parties. But dig some crisps or crackers into a creamy spinach dip and you could be adding 300 calories with just a couple of bites. And that's before you take a sip of the drink that goes with it.

Healthy ways to enjoy

Go for salsa as a dip, either tomato or fruit-based. Houmus (chickpea dip) is a good choice. Most commercially made houmus has about 25 calories per tablespoon. Dip with raw vegetables (carrot, celery, peppers) or with baked tortilla chips rather than with fried ones. Many dips are made with lots of mayonnaise, soured cream and cream cheese. If you are making a dip that calls for mayonnaise, use half mayonnaise and half fat-free yogurt to lower the fat content.

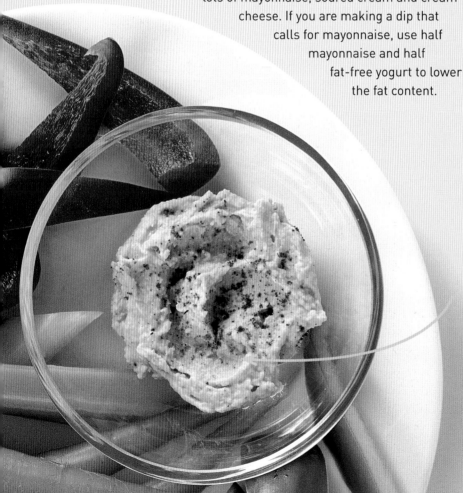

Enjoy your houmus – it's only 25 calories per tablespoon

That 2 tbsp perfect portion of houmus has only 50 calories.

You should always read the serving size labels. Watch them especially on commercially prepared snack foods such as dips. The serving size will probably be 1 or 2 tbsp. If you double that amount when you are eating a snack, you will double the amount of calories, fat and sodium.

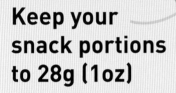

Keep your snack portions to 28g (1oz)

Choose 28g (1oz) baked tortilla chips for around 118 calories.

Dip ideas that won't break the calorie bank

Honey mustard dip (Serves 4)
123g (4½oz) fat-free plain yogurt
2 tbsp honey
3 tbsp Dijon mustard
Place all the ingredients in a jug or bowl and mix together thoroughly with a fork or spoon.

Black bean pâté (Serves 6–8)
425g (15oz) black beans, rinsed and drained
2 tbsp chopped red onion
2 tbsp balsamic vinegar
1 medium garlic clove, peeled and crushed
1 tbsp orange juice
Salt and freshly ground black pepper to taste
Place the black beans in a blender or food processor together with the onion, balsamic vinegar, garlic and orange juice. Blend until thick and smooth. Add salt and pepper to taste.

Dips make great snacks – but choose wisely

eating out

Eating out can be a big portion-plan challenge. When you stop for fast food, you're probably tired or hungry or both, and what do you do? You eat all you order. When you go to a restaurant, you may not know it, but they often have oversized plates that they fill completely. The result? Oversized portions. Then, while you're busy chatting to family and friends, before you know it you've cleaned your plate. When you eat ethnic foods, you need to know the perils of each cuisine so you can make healthy choices. But whether it's fast food, Mexican, Spanish, Japanese, Chinese, Thai, Indian, Italian, French or help-yourself buffets, follow the advice here and you can enjoy eating out and control your portions at the same time.

The perils of eating out

We all enjoy eating out from time to time but this can be a perilous path if you're trying to stick to your Perfect Portion plan. But there's no need to give it up. Simply follow these easy tips and you can enjoy a meal out without having a calorie disaster.

Fast-food sense
Make a fast-food stop into a portion-plan success by ordering carefully. Choose grilled chicken or fish and keep the correct portion size in mind. Go to the salad bar first and half-fill your plate with vegetables. Add just 1 tbsp of dressing.

Eat before you go
Eat a light snack before you go to restaurants or parties so you don't arrive ravenous.

Eat less than you're served
Try to eat only 75 per cent of what's on the plate. A University of Colorado study showed that eating three-quarters of the food normally served on a restaurant plate can save about 300 calories.

Order two starters
Starters in restaurants are now as large as main courses used to be and main courses are, well, enormous! So order two starters instead of a starter and a main course – and save on your calories. Or order a starter and then share a main course.

Remember the 'doggie' bag
If you can't resist eating every bite of an oversized plate, ask for a 'doggie' bag before the meal. When your food arrives, immediately put half of it away and take it home for tomorrow – or for the dog!

Don't go there
Avoid family-style and all-you-can-eat restaurants. They may seem to be offering you a bargain meal, but it's not if you overload on calories.

Follow these tips to avoid a calorie disaster when you eat out

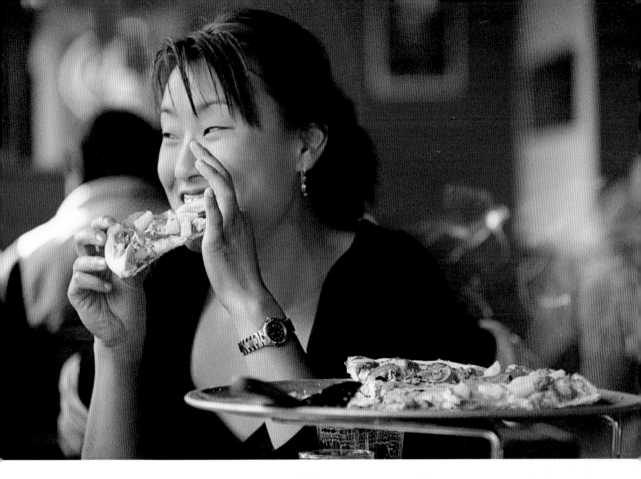

Eating out is a fun and sociable thing to do, but don't eat so much that you regret it the next day. Make careful choices from the menu and keep your portion sizes in mind. It's easy to eat too much when you're chatting to your friends.

Words to avoid

Words like 'large', 'giant' and 'jumbo' are not your friends and should be banned from your vocabulary. Try to steer clear of any dishes whose names contain these wicked words.

Salad days

Eating salads in a restaurant should be fine for your Perfect Portion plan, but not if they're dripping with dressing. Ask for the dressing on the side and dip your pieces of salad into it. Alternatively, scoop out 1 tbsp of dressing, dribble it over and enjoy.

Dessert denial

Most people like dessert but we all know how calorific many of the tastiest desserts are. Giving up dessert is often the hardest thing to do. So what's the answer to this problem? Don't deny yourself. If you do, you may end up eating something worse as soon as you get home. Simply order one dessert for the table so everyone gets a taste. You'll find that just a few bites will satisfy your desire for a sweet ending.

Mexican

Pick up a chicken and bean burrito or order a Chilli Relleno (stuffed pepper) dinner and you may be eating a day's worth of fat that's equivalent to 227g (8oz) of bacon. Refried beans are another disaster. They're usually made with cooked pinto beans mashed with lard, bacon or cheese. A serving of 252g (8¾oz) can add a half day's saturated fat to your portion plan.

Another word of caution – hold back on the second margarita. These drinks can be made with tequila, a sugar and citrus (usually lime juice) mixture, Grand Marnier, Cointreau or Curaçao. A margarita may have as many as 45 calories per 30ml (1fl oz). A 237ml (8fl oz) drink would supply 350 calories and that doesn't count the fried tortilla chips and guacamole you may have with it.

But, Mexican food can be a treat and portion-plan winner providing you make the right choices. Look for chicken fillings and order à la carte if at all possible. This helps to cut down on the beans, guacamole, soured cream and fried tortilla chips that usually come with the meal.

Follow these general guidelines but remember that each restaurant has its own version of these dishes, so it's always best to ask how they are made before you order.

Choices to savour
Fajitas made with grilled or sautéed vegetables and lean meat
• Quesadillas made with a small amount of cheese and lean protein such as chicken or prawns • Burritos made with shredded lettuce, lean beef and a small amount of cheese • Enchiladas made with chicken (avoid if made with lots of cheese and double cream)

Choices to avoid
Sides of soured cream and deep-fried tortilla chips • Refried beans • Chimichangas (deep-fried burrito served with guacamole, cheese and soured cream) • Enchiladas, if softened in a lot of oil • Quesadillas stuffed with cheese • Large bowls of tortilla chips, guacamole and salsa often on the table when you sit down – have the salsa, just a small spoonful of guacamole and no crisps • Pitchers of margaritas or beer

Danger areas
- Lots of cheese
- Dishes with avocado
- Deep-fried foods
- Lots of rice

Spanish

Paella is probably the most famous dish to be found at Spanish restaurants, but it can be a calorie disaster. Eat a plateful and you could be having over 1000 calories. Another danger area can be tapas, those small plates of food that are served in Spanish bars with a drink or that can be combined to make a main meal. The ones to watch are those heavily laden with sausage or cheese, or that are deep-fried.

Another word of caution: watch that pitcher of sangría. With its red wine, orange juice, sugar and possibly orange liqueur, sangría goes down like a cool, fruit drink. But 30ml (1fl oz) can have about 50 calories. A 237ml (8fl oz) glass could add 400 calories to your meal before the food arrives.

Danger areas

- Dishes based on rice
- Dishes with lots of sausage and fatty meats
- Dishes based on deep-fried foods
- Dishes using salt cod (bacalao) for their high salt content

Choices to savour

Ensaladas (various salads – ask for the dressing on the side) • Roasted vegetables and meats (look for the word 'asado' on the menu), such as Verduras Asadas (roasted vegetables) • Gazpacho (cold soup made with tomatoes and vegetables, mostly served as a first course) • Grilled vegetables and meats (look for the words 'a la plancha' on the menu), such as Champiñones a la Plancha (grilled mushrooms), Camarones a la Plancha (grilled shrimp), Calamares a la Plancha (grilled squid) • Most fish or chicken dishes made with tomato or other vegetables • Grilled or roasted meat or seafood, such as Cochinillo Segoviano (roast suckling pig) – ask for a 170g/6oz portion with the fat removed) • Salmon or dorado

Choices to watch

Morcilla (blood sausage) • Chorizo Cantimpalo (Spanish-style sausage) • Manchego, Cabrales or any cheese in more than a 57g (2oz) portion • Deep-fried foods (look for words like 'fritura' or 'frito' on the menu), such as Fritura Mixta de Pescado (mixed deep-fried fish) • Food cooked with a lot of oil (look for words like 'al aceite' or 'al ajillo'), such as Gambas al Ajillo (shrimp cooked in parsley, oil and garlic) • Cochinillo Segoviano (roast suckling pig with skin and fat) • Heavy stews with thick sausages and a lot of potatoes • Dishes based on lots of rice such as Paella or Arroz con Pollo (chicken with rice) • Cortes Grasos del Filete (fatty meats)

Japanese

Talk about Japanese food today and most people think sushi. Seafood, nori (seaweed) and vegetables are healthy ingredients in sushi. A 113g (4oz) sushi serving with nori and rice is about 350 calories. Beware, though. You can eat a double and triple portion without realizing it. And dipping your sushi in soy sauce adds salt to the equation. Also, watch the raw fish. Pregnant women and those with immune disorders should not eat raw fish or shellfish as there's a risk of exposure to parasites and to bacteria such as *Listeria monocytogenes*. For others these risks may be considered minimal, as long as the fish is sushi quality and fresh.

Danger areas

- Sushi with excessive rice
- Large servings of sushi
- Large bowls of rice
- Deep-fried foods

Another thing to watch for is the *sake*. Potent, warm *sake* is very inviting. One or two small servings is fine, but drink more from the attractive little bottle it's served in and you'll be adding about 500 calories to your meal.

As with most Asian dishes, meat and vegetables are a good choice if you stay away from the sugary, salty sauces. Or, make sure you have very little sauce.

Follow these general guidelines but remember that each restaurant has its own version of these dishes, so it's always best to ask how they are made before you order.

Choices to savour

Sushi made with cooked crab, prawns or eel, scrambled egg, tofu or simply vegetables • Sashimi (raw fish dipped in soy sauce, usually flavoured with horseradish) • Miso (fermented soya bean) soup • Teppanyaki dishes (meat, fish or vegetables cooked on an iron griddle) • Sukiyaki dishes (meat and vegetables usually cooked at the table in a shallow pan)

Choices to watch

Tempura (vegetables or seafood coated in batter and deep-fried) • Teriyaki (shellfish or meat with a marinade of soy sauce, sugar and rice wine) with a thick coating of sugary sauce • Yakitori (skewered meat basted with soy sauce, stock, sugar and rice wine) – again watch the sauce

Chinese

Many think that Chinese food with its vegetables and small pieces of meat is more healthy than other ethnic foods. But look at these numbers and then make careful choices. Chinese foods are a blend of sweet and salty flavours. This means they can be loaded with sugar and salt. An order of Lo Mein (boiled noodles) can have as much salt as a large pizza. Even stir-fried vegetables can have over 2000mg sodium – about a day's quota of salt. Many dishes are also high in fat. The popular dish Kung Pao Chicken can have as much as 76g of fat in an average serving. That's more than an entire day's amount. And then there's all that rice and noodles, too.

Danger areas

- Thick sweet and sour sauces
- Large bowls of fried rice
- Deep-fried foods

You can make healthier choices when you're eating a Chinese meal. Start by removing deep-fried batter coatings and, for the least amount of fat, choose stir-fried seafood and vegetables. Eat the meat and vegetables, but leave much of the sauce behind. Plan on a main course that you estimate has about 142g (5oz) of meat, and 300–340g (10½–12oz) of vegetables with 119g (4¼oz) rice. Finally, stay away from dishes based only on rice or noodles.

Follow these general guidelines but remember that each restaurant has its own version of these dishes so it's best to ask how they are made.

Choices to savour

These are good choices to look for: Stir-fried prawns or vegetables
• Steamed vegetables • Steamed brown rice

Choices to watch

Many of these popular dishes can be fine, but here are areas to watch: Fried rice, especially eaten as a main course • Orange Crispy Beef (if coated in batter, try peeling off the batter before eating) • Szechuan Prawns (breaded or deep-fried) • Fried spring rolls • Beef or pork dishes if made with fattier cuts • Sweet and sour dishes thickly battered and with a thick, sugary sauce • Lo Mein • Chow Mein • Dumplings (especially deep-fried) • Chinese spareribs

Thai

On a culinary trip to Bangkok, a Thai friend told me she never cooks real Thai food at home because it takes so much time to properly prepare the ingredients. Perhaps that's why so many go out to restaurants for Thai food. The spiciness and unique blend of flavours have made Thai cooking popular around the world. But among these flavours lurk some problems that can damage your portion plan.

Fortunately, a staple of Thai cuisine is fish and seafood, and soups abound that contain little fat but are packed with flavour. A favourite method of cooking is satay, which offers lean meats cooked without added oil. The streets of Bangkok are filled with street vendors offering these meats cooked over hot coals on skewers. With the information below you can enjoy this popular style of eating guilt-free.

Follow these general guidelines but remember that each restaurant has its own version of these dishes, so it's always best to ask how they are made before you order.

Choices to savour
Dom Yang Gung (hot and sour prawn soup) • Tom Yam Kung (sour prawn soup) • Chicken, fish or lean meat satay with 1 tbsp peanut sauce • Moo Daeng (roasted pork—170g/6oz portion) • Tode Mun Plah (spicy fish cakes) • Yum Neua Yahng (grilled beef salad with chillies and lime • Sam Tum (green papaya salad) • Miang Yuan (soft spring rolls with prawns and fresh mint)

Choices to watch
Kao Pad (fried rice) • Pad Thai (fried noodles, usually with prawns) • Crab Rangoon (pastry wraps stuffed with crab, soft white cheese and spices) • Mee Krob (crispy fried noodles) • Kaeng Keo Wan Kai (green chicken curry or any curries made with thick coconut milk and palm sugar) • Massaman Beef Curry (fatty short ribs, potatoes, coconut and nuts) • Sticky rice in large amounts • Sauces such as Nam Jim Satay (savoury peanut sauce made with coconut cream, sugar and peanuts) and Nahm Jim Gratiem (a nearly caramelized sweet and spicy sauce that is mostly sugar)

Indian

Hot and spicy curries, a wide choice of vegetarian dishes, delicious chutneys and breads that range from thin and crispy to fat and filled – all these make Indian food a treat. Eating in an Indian restaurant, though, can be a portion control disaster as many dishes are based on lots of rice, sauces are often creamy and sweet, ghee (clarified butter) is used for frying and portions can be over-large.

As with all ethnic food, you will make the best choices by knowing your way around the menu. When eating Indian food, it is best to order the rice on the side and take only 119g (4¼oz). Order a side dish of vegetables to go with the main dishes and you'll eat healthily and without breaking your calorie bank.

Follow these general guidelines but remember that each restaurant has its own version of these dishes, so it's always best to ask how they are made before you order.

Choices to savour

Dishes roasted in a tandoori oven (look for the word 'tandoori' on the menu), such as Tandoori Chicken • Dishes made with green vegetables, usually spinach (look for the word 'saag' on the menu), such as Chicken Saag (sautéed spiced chicken and spinach) • Dishes marinated in spices and roasted in a tandoori oven (look for the word 'tikka' on the menu), such as Fish Tikka • Roti (unleavened bread baked in clay oven) • Raita (cucumber, yogurt and herbs side dish)

Choices to watch

Dishes made with a cream sauce and probably also with almonds and cashew nuts (look for the word 'korma' on the menu), such as Lamb Korma • Dishes cooked with rice (look for the word 'biryani' on the menu), such as Lamb Biryani • Dishes with a creamy tomato sauce (look for the word 'masala' on the menu), such as Chicken Tikka Masala • Chutneys add flavour to dishes, but they contain a lot of sugar, so eat them sparingly • Side dishes such as poppadums (crisp bread dried and fried in hot fat) and samosas (deep-fried vegetable/meat stuffed pastry)

Italian

Going out for Italian food can either be a great choice or a disastrous one. Italians love vegetables and there are always plenty to choose from on their menus. Seafood is another Italian favourite. Either of these foods can be healthy choices as long as they aren't swimming in oil.

But, order Calamari Fritti (fried squid rings) as a starter and it could add up to 600 calories – and that's before you eat your dinner. Choose Melanzane alla Parmigiana (aubergine Parmesan) and you could be eating about 1600 calories. Pasta is another food to keep an eye on. A small side dish of about 57–85g (2–3oz) cooked pasta is fine, but watch the large platefuls served as a main course.

Most Italian restaurant dishes will be overloaded with oil or butter. If possible ask if the dish can be cooked in small amount of oil. For marinated vegetables, ask for the dressing on the side or leave most on the plate. Order grilled meat, chicken or fish. If ordering pizza, ask for little or no cheese and plan to share the pizza with others at the table (*see also Portion Distortion Pizza, pages 116–117*).

Follow these general guidelines but remember that each restaurant has its own version of these dishes, so it's always best to ask how they are made before you order.

Choices to savour
Chicken Marsala (go light on the sauce) • Pasta e Fagioli (Pasta and bean soup, small bowl or as a main course) • Vegetable Antipasto (ask for a small portion and dressing on the side) • Minestrone soup • Fish, chicken or meat with two vegetables rather than with pasta

Choices to watch
Veal Parmigianino (breaded veal with tomato sauce and a thick coating of cheese) • Lasagne (eat a very small portion) • Fettuccine Alfredo (noodles with a double cream, egg and cheese sauce) • Linguine with Italian sausages • Spaghetti Carbonara (made with bacon, double cream, eggs, butter and Parmesan cheese) • Frito Misto (a plate of deep-fried mixed seafood) • Osso Bucco (braised veal shank) • Calzone and cannelloni— when stuffed with a lot of cheese

French

While living in France, I enjoyed French cuisine, but wondered why I never gained any weight. I finally realized it was because of the portion sizes and the balanced meals. Meals started with a vegetable such as asparagus as a first course, continued with a small piece of meat, poultry or fish and a small portion of potatoes for the main course. This was followed by a salad. Dessert was usually some fruit and a little cheese. On some occasions we had a sweet dessert. This was a far cry from the creamy sauces and over-loaded plates of French food I was used to in French restaurants in America. So, don't give up on French food, but do plan your portions and selections with care.

To help you limit your calorie and fat intake, ask for 170g (6oz) portions of meats or seafood with the sauce on the side, and order two vegetables instead of creamy potatoes or chips. And though pairing French food with wine is a treat, stick to one glass for women and two for men. A glass of wine should measure 148ml (5fl oz).

Follow these general guidelines but remember that each restaurant has its own version of these dishes, so it's always best to ask how they are made before you order.

Choices to savour
Crudités (platter of raw cut vegetables) • Most vegetables, steamed or blanched and served with a little oil • Ratatouille (tomato, aubergine, courgette) • Clear soups such as Soupe aux Champignons (mushroom) or Potage aux Asperges (asparagus) • Soupe de Poissons (fish soup) • Fish dishes in a light sauce • Moules à la Marinière (mussels)

Choices to watch
Mousses (savoury or sweet) • Pâté or terrines • Veau à la crème (veal in cream sauce) • Sauce Hollandaise (made with eggs and butter) • Beurre Blanc (made with white wine, shallots and butter) • Sauce Béarnaise (made with vinegar, shallots, tarragon, eggs and butter)

Portion distortion: buffet food

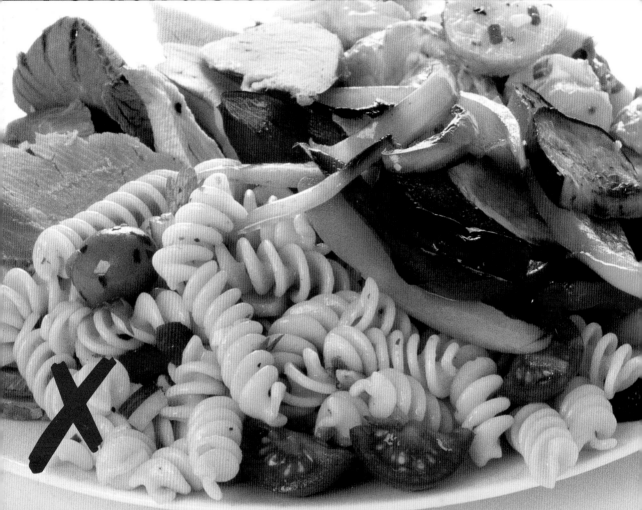

oversize portion

Love buffets and all the choice they offer? How do you decide between juicy roast beef, honey-roasted ham, pasta salad or potato salad? And what about the dessert table? You overload your plate and then go back for seconds. It's a temptation that's hard to resist. But look at this plate. It's got so much food on it that it's hard to tell what you're eating. If your plate tends to look like this, read on and you can mend your ways.

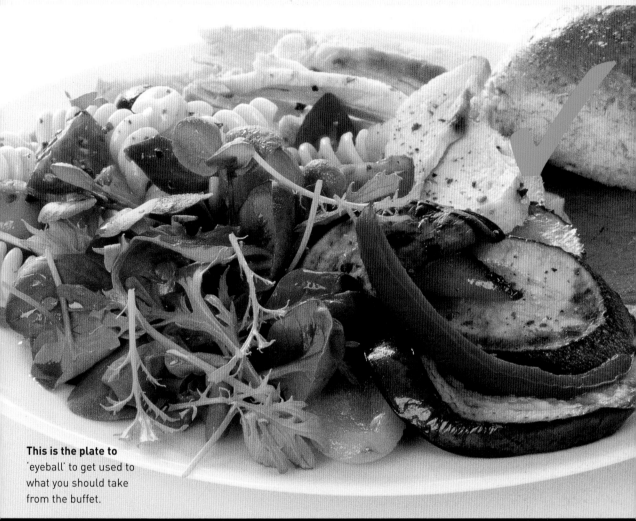

This is the plate to 'eyeball' to get used to what you should take from the buffet.

perfect portion

This healthy plateful has 142g (5oz) lean meat, 162g (5³⁄₄oz) grilled vegetables, 47g (1³⁄₄oz) salad greens, 1 tbsp dressing, 209g (7¹⁄₂oz) pasta salad with vegetables, and 1 small wholemeal roll. At the buffet: concentrate on salad and vegetables; have 78–156g (2³⁄₄–5¹⁄₂oz) pasta, potatoes or other starch; choose fresh fruit for dessert, or a miniature pastry, or a 2.5cm (1in) slice of cake; don't make a second trip.

Nutritional analysis
per plate of buffet food as pictured

653 calories with 36 per cent from fat; **26.3g** fat, of which, **5.9g** saturated fat; **48.3g** protein; **98mg** cholesterol; **1119mg** sodium; **9.6g** fibre

7-day eating plan

Are you tempted by a breakfast of granola, yogurt and almonds or by a creamy cheese omelette and grapefruit? Do you like the sound of mushroom quiche for lunch, or a garlic steak, baked potato and green beans for dinner? My Seven-Day Eating Plan includes all these dishes and more. It epitomizes everything Perfect Portion is about – how to enjoy great, quick-to-make food in portions that won't pile on the weight, and how to eat balanced meals that will help keep you healthy. Each day of the Plan gives you breakfast, lunch and dinner. I also suggest alternative dinners for vegetarians. Make this Seven-Day Eating Plan your blueprint for life. Substitute your favourite foods – in perfect portions, of course! Now you can enjoy the food you like for ever more.

Day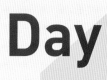

MENU

Note on quantities

All the recipes in this Seven-Day Eating Plan give quantities for approximately 1400 calories a day. If you are very active, you may need about 1800 calories a day. The asterisked quantities below each recipe are for an 1800-calorie day. See page 176 for full nutritional information.

Wholemeal bagel with cream cheese and smoked fish

1400 calorie breakfast per serving: 423 calories
1800 calorie breakfast per serving: 456 calories

Mushroom cheddar crustless quiche and salad

1400 calorie lunch per serving: 407 calories
1800 calorie lunch per serving: 538 calories

Lamb kebabs and brown rice

1400 calorie dinner per serving: 551 calories
1800 calorie dinner per serving: 851 calories

Total day calories: 1381/1845

Breakfast

Wholemeal bagel with cream cheese and smoked fish

1 wholemeal bagel, 7.5cm (3in) in diameter (about 57g/2oz)
1 tbsp reduced-fat cream cheese
85g (3oz)* smoked fish (mackerel, haddock, salmon)
1 medium tomato, sliced
Several lettuce leaves

30g (1oz) bran cereal
118ml (4fl oz) skimmed milk

For 1800 calories
*113g (4oz) smoked fish

Cut the bagel in half and spread both sides with the cream cheese. Top with the smoked fish, tomato and lettuce. Serve the cereal with skimmed milk.

Lunch

Mushroom cheddar crustless quiche and salad

Olive oil spray
27g (1oz)* wholemeal breadcrumbs
35g (1¼oz) sliced mushrooms
57g (2oz)** smoked turkey breast, cut into cubes
1 whole egg
1 egg white
Salt and freshly ground black pepper
28g (1oz) grated, reduced-fat mature Cheddar cheese

For salad
47–55g (1¾–2oz) washed, ready-to-eat salad
1 tbsp reduced-fat oil and vinegar dressing

For 1800 calories
*54g (2oz) wholemeal breadcrumbs
**113g (4oz) smoked turkey breast

Spray a 7.5cm (3in) tartlet tin with olive oil spray. Sprinkle the breadcrumbs on the bottom. Add the mushrooms and turkey breast. Mix 1 whole egg and 1 egg white together, add salt and pepper to taste, and pour over the mushrooms and turkey. Sprinkle the cheese on top and bake in a 180°C (350°F/Gas 4) oven for 20 minutes. Serve with the salad and dressing.

For dessert:1 apple (about the size of a fist or 106g).

Dinner

Lamb kebabs

170g (6oz)* lamb cut from the leg and cut into
    4cm (1½in) cubes
113g (4oz)** courgettes, cut into 2.5cm (1in) slices
½*** medium yellow pepper, cut into 2.5cm (1in)
    pieces
5 cherry or grape tomatoes

For 1800 calories
*227g (8oz) lamb
**227g (8oz) courgettes
***1 medium yellow pepper

Marinate the lamb in 2 tbsp lemon juice, 1 clove crushed garlic and 1 tsp rosemary for 15 minutes while the other ingredients are prepared.

Preheat the grill. Alternate the courgettes, yellow pepper and cherry tomatoes on a metal skewer. Remove the lamb from the marinade and thread another skewer leaving 1cm (½in)

Lean lamb is a great choice – it's low in calories and has only 36% fat

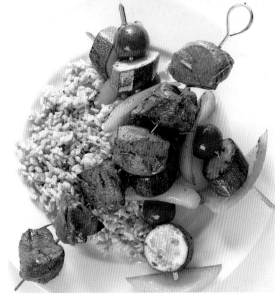

Lamb kebabs and brown rice

between the cubes. Place both on a foil-lined baking tray. Grill the kebabs 15cm (6in) from the heat for 5 minutes, then turn over and grill for another 5 minutes. Serve accompanied by rice (*see below*).

Brown rice
63g (2¼oz)* 10-minute brown rice
2 tsp** olive oil
Salt and freshly ground black pepper

For 1800 calories
*94g (3½oz)10-minute brown rice
**3 tsp olive oil

Follow the packet instructions to cook the rice. Toss with the olive oil and season with salt and pepper to taste. The cooked rice yields may vary by brand. For a 1400-calorie per day menu, serve 146g (5¼oz) of cooked rice. For an 1800-calorie a day menu, serve 260g (9oz) of cooked rice.

Vegetarian dinner suggestion
Instead of the Lamb Kebab. Toss 128g (4¾oz) rinsed and drained red kidney beans and 35g (1¼oz) unsalted almonds with the brown rice.

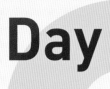

Day 2

MENU

Note on quantities

All the recipes in this Seven-Day Eating Plan give quantities for approximately 1400 calories a day. If you are very active, you may need about 1800 calories a day. The asterisked quantities below each recipe are for an 1800-calorie day. See pages 176–177 for full nutritional information.

Egg scramble, wholemeal toast and tomato juice

1400 calorie breakfast per serving: 320 calories
1800 calorie breakfast per serving: 431 calories

Ham and cheese melt

1400 calorie lunch per serving: 483 calories
1800 calorie lunch per serving: 606 calories

Sole parmesan and broccoli pasta

1400 calorie dinner per serving: 562 calories
1800 calorie dinner per serving: 748 calories

Total day calories: 1365/1784

Breakfast

Microwave egg scramble with wholemeal toast and tomato juice

2 tbsp* grated, reduced-fat Emmenthal cheese
1 whole egg
1** egg white
Salt and freshly ground black pepper
1 slice*** wholemeal toast
177ml (6fl oz) glass low-sodium tomato juice

30g (1oz) bran cereal
118ml (4fl oz) skimmed milk

For 1800 calories
*4 tbsp grated reduced-fat Emmenthal cheese
** 2 egg whites
***2 slices wholemeal toast

Place the grated cheese in a small microwave-safe bowl or ramekin. Add the whole egg, egg white and salt and pepper to taste. Mix well. Cover with kitchen paper and microwave on high for 30 seconds. Remove from the microwave, stir and microwave for 20 seconds.

Alternatively, mix the cheese, egg, egg white and salt and pepper to taste together in a small bowl. Heat a non-stick frying pan over a medium-high heat and scramble the eggs. Stir and serve on a slice of toast. Serve with a 177ml (6fl oz) glass of low-sodium tomato juice. Serve bran cereal with skimmed milk.

Lunch

Ham and cheese melt

43g (1½oz)* or ¼ of a 30cm (12in) wholegrain baguette
olive oil spray
1 medium tomato, sliced
57g (2oz) lean ham
43g (1½oz)** brie or other soft cheese

For 1800 calories

*57g (2oz) or 1/3 of a 30cm (12in) wholegrain baguette
**57g (2oz) brie

Preheat the grill to medium-high. Slice the bread open lengthways and spray with olive oil spray. Toast for 30 seconds, then place the tomato slices on one half together with the ham and then the cheese on top. Toast until the cheese melts. Close with the top half and serve.

For dessert: 1 medium pear.

Dinner

Sole parmesan

1 tsp olive oil
170g (6oz)* sole, grouper, grey mullet, mahi-mahi, or other non-oily fish fillet
63g (2¼oz) low-sodium pasta sauce
**1 tbsp grated Parmesan cheese

For 1800 calories

*227g (8oz) fish fillet
**2 tbsp grated Parmesan cheese

Heat a non-stick frying pan over a medium-high heat and add the olive oil. Add the fish and sauté for 4 minutes. Turn the fish over and sauté for 2 minutes. Spoon the pasta sauce over the fish and sprinkle with Parmesan cheese. Cover with a lid and cook for 2 minutes. Serve with Broccoli Pasta (*see right*).

White fish only contains 156 calories per 170g (6oz) portion

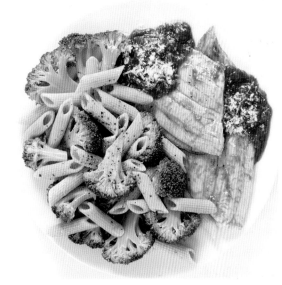

Sole parmesan and broccoli pasta

Broccoli pasta

57g (2oz)* whole-wheat penne pasta
113g (4oz) broccoli florets
2 tsp olive oil
Salt and freshly ground black pepper

For 1800 calories

*113g (4oz) whole-wheat penne pasta

Place a large saucepan filled with 1–4 litres (32–128fl oz) water on to boil. Add the pasta and cook for 5 minutes. Add the broccoli and continue to cook for 3 minutes. Drain and toss with olive oil, then add salt and pepper to taste and serve.

Vegetarian dinner suggestion

Omit the Sole Parmesan. To the pasta add 2 tbsp pine kernels and sprinkle with 1 tbsp Parmesan cheese. Make a salad of 85g (3oz) sliced fennel and 165g (5¾oz) orange segments. Toss with 1 tbsp reduced-fat oil and vinegar dressing.

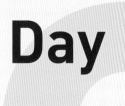

Day 3

MENU

Note on quantities

All the recipes in this Seven-Day Eating Plan give quantities for approximately 1400 calories a day. If you are very active, you may need about 1800 calories a day. The asterisked quantities below each recipe are for an 1800-calorie day. See page 177 for full nutritional information.

Muesli cereal with fruit

1400 calorie breakfast per serving: 374 calories
1800 calorie breakfast per serving: 467 calories

Hamburger and coleslaw

1400 calorie lunch per serving: 514 calories
1800 calorie lunch per serving: 631 calories

Balsamic pork scaloppini and courgette sweet potatoes

1400 calorie dinner per serving: 520 calories
1800 calorie dinner per serving: 695 calories

Total day calories: 1408/1793

Breakfast

Muesli cereal with fruit

41g (1½oz) no-sugar-added muesli cereal
118ml (4fl oz) skimmed milk
62–83g (2¼–3oz) blueberries, strawberries or
    raspberries
1 slice* wholemeal toast
43g (1½oz)** grated, reduced-fat Cheddar cheese

For 1800 calories

* 2 slices wholemeal toast
**57g (2oz) grated, reduced-fat Cheddar cheese

Preheat the grill. Place the muesli in a bowl, add the milk and top with berries. Toast the slice of bread under the grill, add the cheese and grill until the cheese has melted.

Lunch

Hamburger and coleslaw

85g (3oz)* lean minced sirloin
7.5cm (3in) wholemeal hamburger roll,
    about 43g (1½oz)
2 slices tomato
1 tbsp ketchup
60g (2oz) coleslaw

For 1800 calories

*170g (6oz) lean minced sirloin

Preheat the grill. Form the minced sirloin into a burger with your hands. Place the burger on a foil-lined grill rack and grill until desired doneness.
    Split the burger bun in half, add the cooked burger to the base, followed by the tomato slices, ketchup and coleslaw. Cover with the lid and serve.

For dessert: 160g (5¾oz) seedless grapes.

Dinner

Balsamic pork scaloppini

170g (6oz)* pork tenderloin, cut into
    5cm (2in) slices
olive oil spray
59ml (2fl oz) balsamic vinegar
1 tbsp pine kernels
Salt and freshly ground black pepper
1 tbsp chopped parsley (optional)

For 1800 calories
*227g (8oz) pork tenderloin

Remove the fat from the pork tenderloin, then
flatten the slices to about 5mm (¼in) thick. Heat
a non-stick frying pan over a medium-high heat
and spray with olive oil spray. Sauté the pork for
2 minutes on each side. Remove from the pan
and keep warm. Add the balsamic vinegar and
pine kernels to the pan and cook for about 1
minute until the liquid is reduced by half.

Sprinkle the pork with salt and pepper to
taste, spoon the sauce on top, then sprinkle
over the parsley, if using.

Courgette sweet potatoes

142g (5oz)* sweet potato
227g (8oz) courgettes
2 tsp** olive oil
Salt and freshly ground black pepper

For 1800 calories
*227g (8oz) sweet potato
**3 tsp olive oil

Wash and peel the sweet potato and cut into
2.5cm (1in) pieces. Place in a saucepan of cold
water, cover, bring to the boil and cook for 5
minutes. Cut the courgettes into 1cm (½in)
slices and add them to the potatoes. Boil,
uncovered, for 5 minutes, then drain the
vegetables and toss with the olive oil. Season
with salt and pepper to taste and serve.

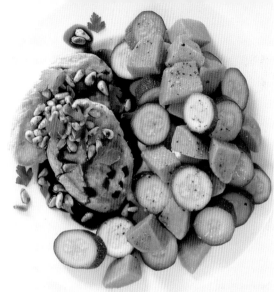

Balsamic pork scaloppini and courgette sweet potatoes

Vegetarian Suggestion
Omit Balsamic Pork Scaloppini and substitute
with Frittata Primavera (*see below*).

Frittata primavera
Olive oil spray
115g (4oz) red onion, sliced
1 medium garlic clove, crushed
½ medium green pepper, sliced,
    about 45g (1½oz)
70g (2½oz) mushrooms, sliced
1 whole egg
2 egg whites
11g (½oz) torn fresh basil
118ml (4fl oz) skimmed milk
Salt and freshly ground black pepper
1 tbsp grated Parmesan cheese

Preheat the grill. Heat a non-stick frying pan
over a medium-high heat and spray with olive oil
spray. Add the onion, garlic, pepper and
mushrooms and sauté for 5 minutes. Mix
together the egg, egg whites, basil and milk.
Add salt and pepper to taste, then pour the egg
mixture into the pan and toss the vegetables to
spread the mixture throughout the pan. Turn the
heat to low and cook for 10 minutes. Sprinkle
Parmesan on top and grill until the top is set.

Day 4

MENU

Note on quantities
All the recipes in this Seven-Day Eating Plan give quantities for approximately 1400 calories a day. If you are very active, you may need about 1800 calories a day. The asterisked quantities below each recipe are for an 1800-calorie day. See page 177 for full nutritional information.

Oatmeal and soft-boiled egg
1400 calorie breakfast per serving: 377 calories
1800 calorie breakfast per serving: 561 calories

Chicken salad with honey yogurt dressing
1400 calorie lunch per serving: 452 calories
1800 calorie lunch per serving: 622 calories

Grilled salmon fillet and asparagus with new potatoes
1400 calorie dinner per serving: 459 calories
1800 calorie dinner per serving: 599 calories

Total day calories: 1288/1782

Breakfast

Oatmeal and soft-boiled egg
41g (1½oz) oatmeal
118ml (4fl oz) skimmed milk
1* large egg
1 slice** rye bread
1 tsp*** olive oil

For 1800 calories
*2 large eggs
**2 slices rye bread
***2 tsp olive oil

Prepare the oatmeal according to the packet instructions using water. Add milk when completed. Cook the egg in a pan of boiling water until soft-boiled. Toast the bread and spread with olive oil. Serve together.

Lunch

Chicken salad with honey yogurt dressing
113g (4oz)* roasted or rotisserie chicken breast
123g (4½oz)** fat-free plain yogurt
3 tbsp*** Dijon mustard
2 tbsp**** honey
100g (3½oz) washed, ready-to-eat mesclun salad

For 1800 calories
*170g (6oz) chicken breast
**184g (6¾oz) yogurt
***4 tbsp Dijon mustard
****3 tbsp honey

Cut the chicken into thin strips. Mix the yogurt, mustard and honey together. Place the salad on a plate, add the dressing and toss with the salad. Arrange the chicken strips on top.

For dessert: 1 medium orange (165g/5¾oz).

Dinner

Grilled salmon fillet and asparagus

Olive oil spray
170g (6oz)* salmon fillet
salt and freshly ground black pepper
½ tbsp chopped fresh or ½ tsp dried dill
227g (8oz) asparagus

For 1800 calories
*227g (8oz) salmon fillet

Preheat the oven grill to medium-high. Line a baking sheet with foil and spray with olive oil spray. Place the salmon fillet on the foil-lined sheet and spray with olive oil spray. Grill the salmon 15cm (6in) from the heat for 10 minutes. To test, insert the point of a knife into the flesh. It should be opaque not translucent. Remove and sprinkle with salt and pepper to taste and dill.

Meanwhile, line another baking sheet with foil and spray with olive oil spray. Cut the woody ends off the asparagus, then arrange in a single layer on the sheet and spray with olive oil spray. Season with salt and pepper to taste. Place on the shelf below the salmon and roast for 5 minutes for thin and 10 minutes for thick. Serve with new potatoes (*see below*).

New potatoes

113g (4oz)* small new potatoes, about ¾in (2cm) in diameter
1 tbsp oil and vinegar dressing
Salt and freshly ground black pepper

For 1800 calories
*142g (5oz) small new potatoes

Salmon is rich in omega-3 fatty acids

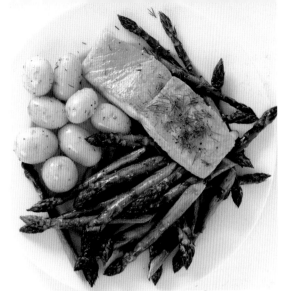

Grilled salmon fillet and asparagus with new potatoes

Wash, but do not peel the potatoes. Place in a saucepan filled with cold water. Cover with a lid and boil for 15 minutes or until cooked through. Toss with 1 tbsp oil and vinegar dressing. Season with salt and pepper to taste.

Vegetarian suggestion

Omit Grilled Salmon Fillet, Asparagus and New Potatoes. Substitute with Potato and White Bean Salad (*see below*).

Potato and white bean salad

113g (4oz) new potatoes, about 2cm (¾in) in diameter
2 tsp olive oil
130g (4¾oz) tinned, rinsed, and drained cannellini beans or other white beans
126g (4½oz) low-sodium pasta sauce
1 medium garlic clove, crushed
1 tsp dried rosemary
½ medium red pepper, sliced
Salt and freshly ground black pepper
2 tbsp grated Parmesan cheese

Wash, but do not peel potatoes. Place them in a saucepan filled with cold water. Cover and boil for 15 minutes or until cooked through. Drain, cut in half, add all the other ingredients and toss well. Garnish with grated Parmesan.

Day 5

MENU

Note on quantities

All the recipes in this Seven-Day Eating Plan give quantities for approximately 1400 calories a day. If you are very active, you may need about 1800 calories a day. The asterisked quantities below each recipe are for an 1800-calorie day. See pages 177–178 for full nutritional information.

Granola cereal with yogurt and almond topping

1400 calorie breakfast per serving: 415 calories
1800 calorie breakfast per serving: 588 calories

Greek salad

1400 calorie lunch per serving: 433 calories
1800 calorie lunch per serving: 519 calories

Chicken provençal and spinach lentils

1400 calorie dinner per serving: 523 calories
1800 calorie dinner per serving: 678 calories

Total day calories: 1371/1785

Breakfast

Granola cereal with yogurt and almond topping

60g (2oz)* low-fat granola cereal
245g (8¾oz)** fat-free, low-sugar, flavoured yogurt
½ tbsp sliced almonds

For 1800 calories
*113g (4oz) granola
**368g (13oz) yogurt

Place the cereal in a bowl and top with the yogurt. Sprinkle the almonds on top and serve.

Lunch

Greek salad

94g (3½oz) washed, ready-to-eat Romaine lettuce
1 medium tomato, cut into quarters
½ medium cucumber sliced, about 60g (2oz)
2 large radishes, sliced, about 27g (1oz)
6 black pitted olives
2 tbsp* reduced-fat oil and vinegar dressing
1 tsp dried oregano
28g (1oz) reduced-fat feta cheese
113g (4oz) ** cooked prawns
½ wholemeal pitta bread

For 1800 calories
* 3 tbsp reduced-fat oil and vinegar dressing
** 170g (6oz) cooked prawns

Place the lettuce, tomato, cucumber, radishes and olives in a bowl. Mix the dressing with the oregano, then add to the salad and toss well. Sprinkle the feta and prawns on top and serve with pitta bread.

Dinner

Chicken provençal

170g (6oz)* boneless, skinless chicken breast
80g (2¾oz) chopped onion
113g (4oz) tinned, chopped tomatoes
1 tsp dried thyme
1 tsp olive oil
2 tsp balsamic vinegar
Salt and freshly ground black pepper

For 1800 calories
*227g (8oz) chicken breast

Heat a non-stick frying pan over a medium-high heat. Add the chicken breast and brown for 2 minutes on each side. Add the onion to the pan and sauté for 2 minutes. Add the tomatoes and thyme, then cover and simmer 5 minutes. Remove from the heat and add the olive oil, balsamic vinegar and salt and pepper to taste. Serve with Spinach Lentils (*see below*).

Spinach lentils

237ml (8fl oz) fat-free, low-sodium chicken stock
48g (1¾oz)* brown lentils
60g (2oz) washed, ready-to-eat spinach
1 tsp** olive oil
Salt and freshly ground black pepper

For 1800 calories
*64g (2¼oz) brown lentils
**2 tsp olive oil

Bring the stock to the boil in a large saucepan. Add the lentils and bring back to the boil. Boil for 20 minutes. Add more stock if the lentils become dry. Add the spinach and stir until wilted. Drain. Add the olive oil and salt and pepper to taste.

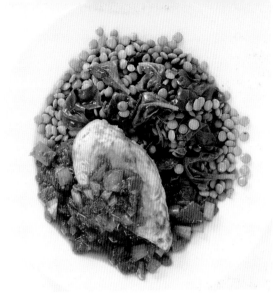

Chicken provençal and spinach lentils

Vegetarian Suggestion
Omit Chicken Provençal and Spinach Lentils and substitute with Spinach and Pimento Lentils and Camembert Salad (*see below*).

Spinach and Pimento Lentils

237ml (8fl oz) fat-free, low-sodium vegetable stock
96g (3½oz) brown lentils
60g (2oz) washed, ready-to-eat spinach
192g (6¾oz) tinned sliced pimento, drained
2 tsp olive oil
Salt and freshly ground black pepper

Bring the stock to the boil in a large saucepan. Add the lentils, bring back to the boil and boil for 20 minutes. Add the spinach and pimento and stir until the spinach is wilted. Drain. Add the olive oil and salt and pepper to taste.

Camembert Salad

94–110g (3½–4oz) washed, ready-to-eat lettuce
1 tbsp reduced-fat oil and vinegar dressing
28g (1oz) Camembert cheese, sliced

Toss the salad with the dressing, then sprinkle the cheese on top and serve.

Day 6

MENU

Note on quantities

All the recipes in this Seven-Day Eating Plan give quantities for approximately 1400 calories a day. If you are very active, you may need about 1800 calories a day. The asterisked quantities below each recipe are for an 1800-calorie day. See page 178 for full nutritional information.

Sunny-side up eggs
1400 calorie breakfast per serving: 349 calories
1800 calorie breakfast per serving: 481 calories

Roast beef wrap
1400 calorie lunch per serving: 495 calories
1800 calorie lunch per serving: 632 calories

Prawn stir-fry and Chinese noodles
1400 calorie dinner per serving: 568 calories
1800 calorie dinner per serving: 706 calories

Total day calories: 1412/1819

Breakfast

Sunny-side up eggs

Olive oil spray
2 whole eggs
1 slice* rye or dark bread

30g (1oz) bran cereal
118ml (4fl oz) skimmed milk

For 1800 calories
*2 slices rye bread
28g (1oz) grated, reduced-fat Cheddar cheese

Spray a non-stick frying pan with olive oil spray and add the eggs. Cook until desired doneness. Serve with toasted bread and a bowl of bran cereal and milk. For a 1800-calorie day, toast the bread with cheese on top to melt.

Lunch

Roast beef wrap

1 tbsp* reduced-fat mayonnaise
1 tbsp** prepared horseradish
20cm (8in) wholemeal tortilla, about 28g (1oz)
113g (4oz)*** lean sliced roast beef
41g (1½oz) tinned sweet pimento, drained
2 Romaine lettuce leaves

For 1800 calories
*1½ tbsp reduced-fat mayonnaise
**1½ tbsp prepared horseradish
***170g (6oz) lean sliced roast beef

Mix the mayonnaise and horseradish together and spread over the tortilla. Arrange the roast beef in a single layer on top and spread the pimento over the beef. Place the lettuce over the pimento and roll up.

For dessert: have an 20cm (8in) banana.

Dinner

Prawn stir-fry

Vegetable oil spray
113g (4oz) trimmed fresh mangetout
58g (2oz) sliced onion
1 medium garlic clove, crushed
1 tbsp chopped fresh ginger or ½ tsp ground
    ginger
170g (6oz)* peeled prawns
2 tbsp low-sodium soy sauce
1 tbsp water
2 tsp toasted or plain sesame oil

For 1800 calories
*227g (8oz) peeled prawns

Heat a wok or frying pan over a high heat and spray with vegetable oil spray. Add the mangetout and onion and stir-fry for 2 minutes. Add the garlic, ginger and prawns and stir-fry for another 2 minutes. In a small bowl, mix the low-sodium soy sauce and water together. Add to the wok and toss for 1 minute. Remove the wok from the heat, add the sesame oil and toss well. Serve with Chinese Noodles (*see right*).

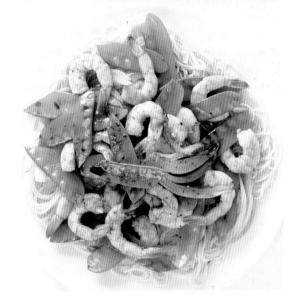

Prawn stir-fry and Chinese noodles

Chinese noodles

57g (2oz)* steamed or fresh Chinese noodles
    (dried angel hair noodles can be substituted)
1 tsp toasted or plain sesame oil

For 1800 calories
*85g (3oz) Chinese noodles

Bring a large saucepan filled with water to the boil. Add the noodles, then bring back to the boil and drain immediately, reserving 1 tbsp water. Toss noodles with the reserved water and sesame oil. Place the noodles on a plate and serve the Prawn Stir-fry on top.

Vegetarian suggestion
Omit the prawns in the stir-fry and substitute 170g (6oz) firm tofu, drained and cut into cubes.

Delicious prawn stir-fry gives you good-quality protein and, as there's no buttery sauce, it's low in saturated fat

Day 7

MENU

Note on quantities

All the recipes in this Seven-Day Eating Plan give quantities for approximately 1400 calories a day. If you are very active, you may need about 1800 calories a day. The asterisked quantities below each recipe are for an 1800-calorie day. See page 178 for full nutritional information.

Breakfast cheese omelette

1400 calorie breakfast per serving: 350 calories
1800 calorie breakfast per serving: 449 calories

Open-faced turkey sandwich

1400 calorie lunch per serving: 485 calories
1800 calorie lunch per serving: 547 calories

Garlic steak dinner and dessert

1400 calorie dinner per serving: 569 calories
1800 calorie dinner per serving: 763 calories

Total day calories: 1404/1759

Breakfast

Breakfast cheese omelette

1* whole egg
2 egg whites
Salt and freshly ground black pepper
1 tsp rapeseed oil
2 tbsp** grated, reduced-fat Cheddar cheese
2 slices toasted wholegrain bread

½ medium grapefruit, 10cm (4in) in diameter

For 1800 calories
*2 whole eggs
**4 tbsp grated cheese

Preheat the oven to 200°C (400°F/Gas 6). Mix the whole egg and egg whites together and season with salt and pepper to taste. Heat the rapeseed oil in a small non-stick frying pan with an ovenproof handle over a medium-high heat. Pour the egg mixture into the pan and let it set for 1 minute. Sprinkle the cheese on top and place the pan in the oven for 3 minutes or until the eggs are set to desired consistency. Serve with wholegrain bread. Serve half a grapefruit.

Lunch

Open-faced turkey sandwich

1 tbsp mayonnaise
1 tbsp fat-free plain yogurt
2 slices multigrain bread
¼ medium cucumber, thinly sliced
113g (4oz) sliced cooked turkey breast
1 tbsp fresh chopped dill or 1 tsp dried dill

For 1800 calories
*170g (6oz) sliced turkey breast

Mix the mayonnaise and yogurt together. Spread a thin layer over the bread, leaving the remaining sauce for the topping. Arrange the cucumber on the bread and then add the turkey slices. Place the remaining mayonnaise sauce on top and sprinkle with dill.

For dessert: 1 medium mango cut into cubes.

Dinner

Garlic steak

1 tsp butter
1 medium garlic clove, crushed
170g (6oz)* sirloin, skirt or flank
Salt and freshly ground black pepper

For 1800 calories
*227g (8oz) steak

Mix the butter and garlic together until smooth. Heat a non-stick frying pan over a medium-high heat. Remove the visible fat from the steak and place in the pan. Brown for 1 minute, then turn and brown for another minute, seasoning with salt and pepper to taste on the cooked sides. Place the butter mixture on the steak and cook for another 2 minutes. A meat thermometer should read 63°C (145°F) for rare or 71°C (160°F) for medium. Serve with Baked Potato and Green Beans (*see below*).

Baked potato

113g (4oz)* red potato
1 tbsp** reduced-fat soured cream
1 tbsp*** chopped fresh chives, or 1 tsp dried

For 1800 calories
*227g (8oz) red potato
**2 tbsp reduced-fat soured cream
***2 tbsp chopped fresh chives, or 2 tsp dried

Preheat the oven to 220°C (425°F/Gas 7). Wash but do not peel potato. Pierce the skin in several places to let the steam escape. Microwave on high 1 minute, remove and place in the oven for

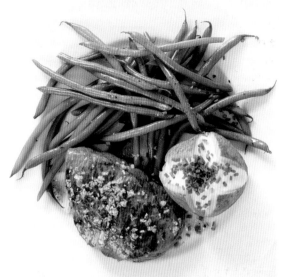

Garlic steak with baked potato and green beans

20 minutes. Alternatively, bake in the oven for 40 minutes. Remove from the oven and cut 2 short slashes, one crossways and one lengthways and squeeze the potato to open. Add soured cream and sprinkle chives on top.

Green beans

113g (4oz) trimmed green beans
½ tsp olive oil
Salt and freshly ground black pepper

Place the green beans in a microwave-safe bowl. Microwave on high 1½ minutes. Alternatively, bring a small saucepan filled with water to the boil. Add the beans, bring back to the boil and cook for 5 minutes. Drain and place in a bowl. Toss with olive oil and season with salt and pepper to taste.

Raspberry sorbet

Serve 88g (3oz) raspberry sorbet for dessert.

Vegetarian Dinner Suggestion

Substitute 227g (8oz) sliced Portobello mushrooms for the steak. Sauté with 1 tsp butter and 1 crushed garlic clove for 5 minutes. Sprinkle 43g (1½oz) blue cheese on top and cover with the pan lid to melt the cheese.

Nutritional analysis for the Seven-Day Eating Plan

Use the following guide to show you the nutritional value of all the meals in my Seven-Day Eating Plan, whether you are following the 1400- or the 1800-calorie-a-day plan.

Day 1

1400 calorie day breakfast per serving: 423 calories (20 per cent from fat), 9.5g fat (4.3g saturated, 0.3g monounsaturated), 39mg cholesterol, 31.1g protein, 69.1g carbohydrates, 18.2g fibre, 1207mg sodium.

1800 calorie day breakfast per serving: 456 calories (21 per cent from fat), 10.8g fat (4.6g saturated, 0.3g monounsaturated), 46mg cholesterol, 36.2g protein, 69.1g carbohydrates, 18.2g fibre, 1429mg sodium.

1400 calorie day lunch per serving: 407 calories (32 per cent from fat), 14.3g fat (3.8g saturated, 3.0g monounsaturated), 257mg cholesterol, 35.4g protein, 35.2g carbohydrates, 6.5g fibre, 539mg sodium.

1800 calorie day lunch per serving: 538 calories (26 per cent from fat), 15.8g fat (4.2g saturated, 3.6g monounsaturated), 295mg cholesterol, 51.8g protein, 48.1g carbohydrates, 8.4g fibre, 717mg sodium.

1400 calorie day dinner per serving: 551 calories (33 per cent from fat), 20.1g fat (4.9g saturated, 10.9g monounsaturated), 108mg cholesterol, 41.4g protein, 51.9g carbohydrates, 7.3g fibre, 122mg sodium.

1800 calorie day dinner per serving: 851 calories (31 per cent from fat), 29.1g fat (6.9g saturated, 5.8g monounsaturated), 144mg cholesterol, 57.9g protein, 91.1g carbohydrates, 12.1g fibre, 164mg sodium.

Vegetarian dinner 1400 calorie day per serving: 571 calories (37 per cent from fat), 23.6g fat (2.7g saturated, 14.9g monounsaturated), 0mg cholesterol, 18.8g protein, 76.6g carbohydrates, 18.3g fibre, 276mg sodium.

Day 2

1400 calorie day breakfast per serving: 320 calories (23 per cent from fat), 8.4g fat (2.4g saturated, 2.6g monounsaturated), 221mg cholesterol, 24.0g protein, 52.0g carbohydrates, 16.3g fibre, 468mg sodium.

1800 calorie day breakfast per serving: 431 calories (21 per cent from fat), 10.2g fat (3.2g saturated, 3.3g monounsaturated), 226mg cholesterol, 34.1g protein, 65.7g carbohydrates, 18.2g fibre, 657mg sodium.

1400 calorie day lunch per serving: 483 calories (30 per cent from fat), 16.0g fat (8.3g saturated, 4.8g monounsaturated), 70mg cholesterol, 25.9g protein, 62.9g carbohydrates, 8.3g fibre, 1175mg sodium.

1800 calorie day lunch per serving: 606 calories (31 per cent from fat), 20.6g fat (10.9g saturated, 6.2g monounsaturated), 84mg cholesterol, 31.4g protein, 77.5g carbohydrates, 9.3g fibre, 1399mg sodium.

1400 calorie day dinner per serving: 562 calories (30 per cent from fat), 18.6g fat (3.5g saturated, 11.0g monounsaturated), 64mg cholesterol, 50.2g protein, 52.94g carbohydrates, 4.7g fibre, 252mg sodium.

1800 calorie day dinner per serving: 748 calories (26 per cent from fat), 21.3g fat (4.7g saturated, 11.6g monounsaturated), 88mg cholesterol, 68.1g protein, 76.0g carbohydrates, 4.8g fibre, 652mg sodium.

Vegetarian dinner 1400 calorie day per serving: 588 calories (38 per cent from fat), 24.6g fat (4.2g saturated, 11.6g monounsaturated), 4mg cholesterol, 21.4g protein, 81.1g carbohydrates, 11.9g fibre, 293mg sodium.

Day 3

1400 calorie day breakfast per serving: 374 calories (17 per cent from fat), 6.9g fat (2.6g saturated, 2.7g monounsaturated), 12mg cholesterol, 21.5g protein, 60.0g carbohydrates, 6.9g fibre, 478mg sodium.

1800 calorie day breakfast per serving: 467 calories (18 per cent from fat), 9.1g fat (3.5g saturated, 3.4g monounsaturated), 15mg cholesterol, 27.7g protein, 73.2g carbohydrates, 8.8g fibre, 713mg sodium.

1400 calorie day lunch per serving: 514 calories (31 per cent from fat), 17.6g fat (4.3g saturated, 2.5g monounsaturated), 64mg cholesterol, 25.1g protein, 69.0g carbohydrates, 6.8g fibre, 711mg sodium.

1800 calorie day lunch per serving: 631 calories (31 per cent from fat), 21.9g fat (6.2g saturated, 4.3g monunsaturated), 118mg cholesterol, 43.3g protein, 69.0g carbohydrates, 6.8g fibre, 768mg sodium.

1400 calorie day dinner per serving: 520 calories (37 per cent from fat), 21.2g fat (4.2g saturated, 10.9g monounsaturated), 108mg cholesterol, 43.0g protein, 42.7g carbohydrates, 7.4g fibre, 191mg sodium.

1800 calorie day dinner per serving: 695 calories (36 per cent from fat), 27.7g fat (5.5g saturated, 15.1g monounsaturated), 144mg cholesterol, 56.1g protein, 58.3g carbohydrates, 9.7g fibre, 261mg sodium.

Vegetarian dinner 1400 calorie day per serving: 558 calories (32 per cent from fat), 19.8g fat (4.5g saturated, 9.1g monounsaturated), 220mg cholesterol, 29.2g protein, 70.4g carbohydrates, 11.8g fibre, 342mg sodium.

Day 4

1400 calorie day breakfast per serving: 377 calories (33 per cent from fat), 13.7g fat (3.1g saturated, 5.8g monounsaturated), 216mg cholesterol, 18.2g protein, 46.5g carbohydrates, 5.9g fibre, 275mg sodium.

1800 calorie day breakfast per serving: 561 calories (39 per cent from fat), 24.4g fat (5.5g saturated, 11.4g monounsaturated), 429mg cholesterol, 27.1g protein, 60.0g carbohydrates, 7.8g fibre, 486mg sodium.

1400 calorie day lunch per serving: 452 calories (7 per cent from fat), 3.5g fat (0.7g saturated, 1.4g monounsaturated), 67mg cholesterol, 38.6g protein, 71.3g carbohydrates, 7.8g fibre, 681mg sodium.

1800 calorie day lunch per serving: 622 calories (7 per cent from fat), 4.8g fat (0.9g saturated, 1.9g monounsaturated),100mg cholesterol, 55.8g protein, 94.5g carbohydrates, 8.3g fibre, 933mg sodium.

1400 calorie day dinner per serving: 459 calories (43 per cent from fat), 22.1g fat (3.6g saturated, 6.0g monounsaturated), 96mg cholesterol, 39.2g protein, 27.0g carbohydrates, 4.3g fibre, 81mg sodium.

1800 calorie day dinner per serving: 599 calories (39 per cent from fat), 26.0g fat (4.2g saturated, 7.2g monounsaturated), 128mg cholesterol, 54.3g protein, 39.7 carbohydrate; 7.6g fibre, 110mg sodium.

Vegetarian dinner 1400 calorie day per serving: 520 calories (30 per cent from fat), 17.5g fat (4.1g saturated, 8.7g monounsaturated), 8mg cholesterol, 22.0g protein, 73.9g carbohydrates, 15.6g fibre, 717mg sodium.

Day 5

1400 calorie day breakfast per serving: 415 calories (20 per cent from fat), 9.3g fat (1.4g saturated, 5.3g monounsaturated), 5mg cholesterol, 21.1g protein, 64.9g carbohydrates, 4.8g fibre, 324mg sodium.

1800 calorie day breakfast per serving: 588 calories (17 per cent from fat), 10.9g fat (1.8g saturated, 6.1g monounsaturated), 8mg cholesterol, 30.4g protein, 96.2g carbohydrates, 6.5g fibre, 486mg sodium.

1400 calorie day lunch per serving: 433 calories (35 per cent from fat), 17.0g fat (5.7g saturated, 2.8g monounsaturated), 197mg cholesterol, 35.1g protein, 38.4g carbohydrates, 9.1g fibre, 1132mg sodium.

1800 calorie day lunch per serving: 519 calories (35 per cent from fat), 20.2g fat (6.1g saturated, 2.9g monounsaturated), 283mg cholesterol, 46.7g protein, 40.2g carbohydrates, 9.3g fibre, 1330mg sodium.

1400 calorie day dinner per serving: 523 calories (22 per cent from fat), 12.7g fat (2.1g saturated, 7.4g monounsaturated), 96mg cholesterol, 57.9g protein, 46.3g carbohydrates, 10g fibre, 745mg sodium.

1800 calorie day dinner per serving: 678 calories (24 per cent from fat), 18.2g fat (2.9g saturated, 11.0g monounsaturated), 128mg cholesterol, 74.8g protein, 55.4g carbohydrates, 11.3g fibre, 782mg sodium.

Vegetarian dinner 1400 calorie day per serving: 597 calories (32 per cent from fat), 21.2g fat (6.3g saturated, 9.2g monounsaturated), 20mg cholesterol, 35.4g protein, 72.7g carbohydrates, 17.8g fibre, 443mg sodium.

Day 6
1400 calorie day breakfast per serving: 349 calories (36 per cent from fat), 13.9g fat (3.7g saturated, 4.3g monounsaturated), 429mg cholesterol, 21.4g protein, 46.4g carbohydrates, 14.9g fibre, 536mg sodium.

1800 calorie day breakfast per serving: 481 calories (32 per cent from fat), 17.0g fat (5.1g saturated, 5.3g monounsaturated), 435mg cholesterol, 31.0g protein, 62.2g carbohydrates, 16.8g fibre, 921mg sodium.

1400 calorie day lunch per serving: 495 calories (29 per cent from fat), 15.8g fat (4.6g saturated, 1.5g monounsaturated), 98mg cholesterol, 38.0g protein, 52.1g carbohydrates, 7.4g fibre, 392mg sodium.

1800 calorie day lunch per serving: 632 calories (32 per cent from fat), 22.6g fat (6.6g saturated 2.2g monounsaturated), 146mg cholesterol, 54.6g protein, 53.6g carbohydrates, 7.7g fibre, 512mg sodium.

1400 calorie day dinner per serving: 568 calories (28 per cent from fat), 17.8g fat (2.8g saturated, 10.8g monounsaturated), 267mg cholesterol, 47.7g protein, 53.8g carbohydrates, 5.4g fibre, 1436mg sodium.

1800 calorie day dinner per serving: 706 calories (25 per cent from fat), 19.3g fat (3.1g saturated, 11.1g monounsaturated), 358mg cholesterol, 62.7g protein, 69.3g carbohydrates, 5.9g fibre, 1577mg sodium.

Vegetarian dinner 1400 calorie day per serving: 520 calories (40 per cent from fat), 23.0g fat (3.4g saturated, 12.2g monounsaturated), 9mg cholesterol, 26.9g protein, 55.4g carbohydrates, 6.0g fibre, 1196mg sodium.

Day 7
1400 calorie day breakfast per serving: 350 calories (33 per cent from fat), 13.0g fat (3.3g saturated, 6.5g monounsaturated), 216mg cholesterol, 22.6g protein, 36.5g carbohydrates, 3.9g fibre, 455mg sodium.

1800 calorie day breakfast per serving: 449 calories (38 per cent from fat), 19.0g fat (5.5g saturated, 8.7g monounsaturated), 432mg cholesterol, 32.3g protein, 37.4g carbohydrates, 3.9g fibre, 605mg sodium.

1400 calorie day lunch per serving: 485 calories (26 per cent from fat), 14.2g fat (2.5g saturated, 4.4g monounsaturated), 84mg cholesterol, 35.2g protein, 57.1g carbohydrates, 7.3g fibre, 376mg sodium.

1800 calorie day lunch per serving: 547 calories (24 per cent from fat), 14.4g fat (2.6g saturated, 4.4g monounsaturated), 122mg cholesterol, 48.9g protein, 57.1g carbohydrates, 7.3g fibre, 406mg sodium.

1400 calorie day dinner per serving: 569 calories (27 per cent from fat), 16.8g fat (7.0g saturated, 6.2g monounsaturated), 120mg cholesterol, 41.3 g protein, 63.5g carbohydrates, 6.3g fibre, 173mg sodium.

1800 calorie day dinner per serving: 763 calories (26 per cent from fat), 22.0g fat (8.4g saturated, 8.4g monounsaturated), 156mg cholesterol, 56.4g protein, 85.1g carbohydrates, 7.8g fibre, 201mg sodium.

Vegetarian dinner 1400 calorie day per serving: 545 calories (35 per cent from fat), 21.0g fat (12.1g saturated, 2.8g monounsaturated), 49mg cholesterol, 21.0g protein, 74.5g carbohydrates, 8.9g fibre, 681mg sodium.

Shopping list for the Seven-Day Eating Plan

Use my shopping list below to help you plan your shopping for the Seven-Day Eating Plan. If you are following the 1800-calorie-a-day plan, the * indicates the quantities you need. If you are cooking the vegetarian alternative dinners, refer to the vegetarian substitutions list on page 180.

Dairy
- Brie or other soft cheese (43g/ 1½oz needed, *57g/2oz needed)
- Butter (57g/2oz needed)
- Cheddar cheese, reduced-fat, grated (85g/3oz needed, *142g/5oz needed)
- Cream cheese, reduced-fat (28g/1oz needed)
- Eggs (10 needed, *13 needed)
- Emmenthal cheese, reduced-fat, grated (14g/¹/₂oz, *28g/1oz needed)
- Feta cheese, reduced-fat (28g/ 1oz needed)
- Parmesan cheese, grated (1 tbsp needed, *2 tbsp needed)
- Skimmed milk (473ml/1 pint)
- Soured cream, reduced-fat (1 small carton)
- Yogurt, fat-free, low-sugar, flavoured (245g/8³/₄oz needed, *368g/13oz needed)
- Yogurt, fat-free plain (154g/5oz, *205/7oz needed)

Deli
- Beef, roast, lean, sliced (113g/4oz, *170g/6oz)
- Chicken breast, roasted or rotisserie (113g/4oz, *170g/6oz)
- Coleslaw (60g/2oz)
- Ham, lean, sliced (57g/2oz)
- Turkey breast, cooked, sliced (113g/4oz, *6oz/170g)
- Turkey breast, smoked, cut into cubes (57g/2oz, *113g/4oz)

Meat
- Chicken breast, boneless, skinless (170g/6oz, *227g/8oz)
- Lamb cut from the leg and cut into 4cm (1½in) cubes (170g/6oz, *227g/8oz)
- Pork tenderloin (170g/6oz, *227g/8oz)
- Sirloin, lean, ground (85g/3oz, *170g/6oz)
- Sirloin, skirt or flank (170g/6oz, *227g/8oz)

Seafood
- Prawns, cooked (113g/4oz, *170g/6oz)
- Prawns, raw and peeled (170g/6oz, *227g/8oz)
- Salmon fillet (170g/6oz, *227g/8oz)
- Smoked fish – mackerel, haddock or salmon (85g/3oz, *113g/4oz)
- Sole, grouper, red mullet, mahi-mahi or other white fish fillet (170g/6oz, *227g/8oz)

Bread
- Multigrain bread (1 small loaf, 2 slices needed – can substitute wholemeal)
- Rye bread (2 slices needed, *4 slices needed – can substitute wholemeal)
- Wholegrain baguette (about 43g/1½oz needed, *57g/2oz needed)
- Wholemeal bagel (1 x 7.5cm/3in in diameter, 57g/2oz)
- Wholemeal bread (1 small loaf)
- Wholemeal hamburger roll (1 x 7.5cm/3in in diameter, 43g/1½oz needed)
- Wholemeal pitta bread (½ pitta)
- Wholemeal tortilla (1 x 20cm/8in, about 28g/1oz)

Grocery
- Almonds, sliced (½ tbsp needed)
- Balsamic vinegar (1 small bottle)
- Black olives, pitted (1 small container/can)
- Bran cereal (1 box, look for 13g fibre per serving)
- Brown lentils (1 small packet)
- Brown rice 10-minute (1 packet)
- Chicken stock, fat-free, low-sodium (237ml/8fl oz needed)
- Chinese noodles, steamed or

fresh – dried angel hair noodles can be substituted (57g/2oz needed, *85g/3oz needed)
- Dijon mustard (1 jar)
- Granola cereal, low-fat (1 box)
- Honey (1 small jar)
- Horseradish, prepared (1 small bottle)
- Ketchup (1 small bottle)
- Mayonnaise (1 small bottle)
- Mayonnaise, reduced-fat (1 small bottle)
- Muesli cereal, no-sugar added (1 packet)
- Oatmeal (1 small packet)
- Olive oil (1 small bottle)
- Olive oil spray
- Oregano, dried (1 small jar)
- Pasta sauce, low-sodium (1 jar/can)
- Pimento, sweet, sliced (1 jar/can)
- Pine kernels (1 tbsp needed)
- Rapeseed oil (1 small bottle)
- Reduced-fat oil and vinegar dressing (1 small bottle)
- Sesame oil, toasted or plain (1 small bottle)
- Soy sauce, low-sodium (1 small bottle)
- Thyme, dried (1 small container)
- Tomato juice, low-sodium (177ml/6fl oz needed)
- Tomatoes, canned, chopped (113g/4oz needed)
- Wholemeal breadcrumbs (1 small container)
- Wholemeal penne pasta (57g/2oz needed, *113g/4oz needed)

Frozen
- Raspberry sorbet (1 small container)

Produce
Vegetables
- Asparagus (227g/8oz)
- Broccoli florets (113g/4oz)
- Chives (1 small bunch or substitute

1 pack freeze-dried chives)
- Courgettes (340g/12oz, *454g/16oz)
- Cucumber (1 medium)
- Dill (1 small bunch or substitute 1 pack freeze-dried dill)
- Garlic (1 head)
- Ginger, fresh (1 small piece or substitute 1 pack ground ginger)
- Green beans (113g/4oz)
- Green pepper (1 medium)
- Mangetout (113g/4oz)
- Mushrooms, sliced (about 35g/1¼oz needed)
- Onion (1 medium)
- Parsley, (optional) (1 small bunch)
- Potatoes, new (113g/4oz *142g/5oz)
- Potatoes, red (113g/4oz, *227g/8oz)
- Potato, sweet (142g/5oz, *227g/8oz)
- Radishes (1 small bunch, 2 needed)
- Red onion (1 medium)
- Romaine lettuce, washed, ready-to-eat (1 x 283g/10oz bag)
- Salad, washed, ready-to-eat, (1 x 283g/10oz bag)
- Salad, mesclun, washed, ready-to-eat (1 x 283g/10oz bag)
- Spinach, washed, ready-to-eat (1 x 283g/10oz bag)
- Tomatoes (4 medium)
- Tomatoes, cherry or grape (5 needed)
- Yellow pepper (1 medium)
Fruit
- Apple (1 medium)
- Banana (1 x 20cm/8in)
- Blueberries, strawberries or raspberries (1 small container)
- Grapefruit (1 medium)
- Grapes, seedless (160g/5¾oz)
- Mango (1 medium)
- Orange (1 medium)
- Pear (1 medium)

Vegetarian substitutions

Day 1: Substitute 1 small pack almonds, 1 small can red kidney beans for the ingredients in the Lamb kebab recipe

Day 2: Substitute 1 small pack pine nuts, 1 tbsp Parmesan cheese, 1 small bulb fennel, 1 orange for the ingredients in the Sole Parmesan recipe

Day 3: Substitute 1 red onion, 1 clove garlic, 1 medium green pepper, 1 small pack fresh mushrooms, 3 eggs, 1 small bunch basil, 1 tbsp Parmesan cheese for the ingredients in the Balsamic pork recipe

Day 4: Substitute 113g (4oz) small new potatoes, 1 can cannellini or other white beans, 1 clove garlic, 1 small bottle dried rosemary, 1 medium red pepper, 2 tbsp Parmesan cheese for the ingredients in the Grilled salmon, asparagus and New potatoes recipes

Day 5: Substitute 237ml (8fl oz) fat-free, low-sodium vegetable broth, 1 small packet brown lentils, 1 jar/can pimento, 1 small bag washed, ready-to-eat spinach, 1 small bag washed, ready-to-eat lettuce, 1 small pack camembert cheese for the ingredients in the Chicken provençal and Spinach lentils recipes

Day 6: Substitute 170g (6oz) firm tofu for the shrimp

Day 7: Substitute 227g (8oz) Portobello mushrooms and 1 small pack blue cheese for the steak

Directory of Perfect Portion foods

Want to find out quickly how much you can eat of a favourite food? The directory below is your easy-to-use reference list for all the foods in Perfect Portion. It shows you at a glance what's OK to choose and how much, which foods you need to watch, and which you should avoid. This doesn't mean you should *never* eat "choices to avoid" – a deviation once in a while is OK, especially once you've mastered the portion guidelines.

Key:
✓ = choices to savour
✳ = choices to watch
✗ = choices to avoid (no weights/ sizes given)

A
✓ almonds, as snack, 28g (1oz), *see* p.140
✳ apple juice, unsweetened, 177ml (6fl oz), *see* pp.91, 132

B
✳ bacon, back, uncooked, 170g (6oz), *see.* p39
bagel, *see* Portion distortion pp.108–109
beef
  ✳ brisket, uncooked, 170g (6oz), *see* p.35
  ✓ chuck steak, uncooked, 170g (6oz), *see* p.35
  ✓ fillet steak, uncooked,170g (6oz), *see* p.35
  ✓ flank steak, uncooked, 170g (6oz), *see* p.35
  minced
    ✗ lean, *see* p.35
    ✓ extra-lean, uncooked, 170g (6oz), *see* p.35
  ✓ porterhouse, uncooked, 170g (6oz), *see* p.35

✗ prime rib joint, *see* p.35
✳ rib-eye steak, uncooked, 170g (6oz), *see* p.35
✓ roast, lean, slices, 113g (4oz), lunch portion, *see* p.45
  ✳ rump steak, uncooked, 170g (6oz), *see* p.35
✗ salt, *see* p.45
✓ sirloin steak, uncooked, 6oz (170g), *see* p.35
✳ skirt, uncooked, 170g (6oz), *see* p.35
✓ T-bone, uncooked, 170g (6oz), *see* p.35
✓ topside, uncooked, 170g (6oz), *see* p.35
beer, *see* pp.136–7
✓ regular, 355ml (12fl oz)
✓ light, 355ml (12fl oz)
bread
  ✳ baguette, 28g (1oz), *see* p.97
  ✳ English muffin, wholemeal, half, *see* p.61
garlic, *see* p.97
  ✗ bought or restaurant
  ✳ home-made, *see* recipe on p.97
pitta, *see* pp.95, 96
  ✳ white, 6in (15cm)
  ✓ wholemeal, 6in (15cm)
✓ rye bread, 1–2 slices/28–57g (1–2oz), *see* p.96
✓ tortilla, flour, 15cm (6in), *see* p.96

✗ white, *see* p.96
✓ wholegrain, 1–2 slices/28–57g (1–2oz), *see* p.95
✓ wholemeal, 1–2 slices/28–57g (1–2oz), *see* pp.94, 95
breakfast cereals, *see* pp.110–111
  ✓ granola, low-fat, 60g (2oz)
  ✓ high-fibre, bran or whole grains, about 30g (1oz)
  ✓ muesli, low-fat, about 60g (2oz)
  ✓ oatmeal, about 30g (1oz)
✳ brownie, 2.5cm (1in) square, *see* p.126
✓ buckwheat, 126g (4½oz), *see* p.113
buffet food, *see* Portion distortion, pp.158-9
✓ bulgur wheat, 182g (6½oz), *see* pp.112–13
✳ butter, 1 tsp, *see* pp.62, 63

C
cakes, *see* Desserts
cereals, breakfast, *see* Breakfast cereals
cheese, *see* pp.64–5
  ✓ cheddar, reduced-fat, 43–57g (1½–2oz)
  ✓ cottage cheese, reduced-fat, 43–57g (1½–2oz)
  ✓ cream cheese, reduced-fat, 43–57g (1½–2oz)
  ✓ Emmenthal, reduced-fat,

43–57g (1½–2oz)

✗ full-fat, any

✗ mozzarella, deep-fried

✓ ricotta, reduced-fat, 43–57g (1½–2oz)

chicken

✓ breast, boneless, skinless, uncooked, 170g (6oz), see p.42

✗ breast with skin and fat, see p.42

✓ breast, oven-roasted, slices, 113g (4oz), lunch portion, see p.45

✗ dark meat with skin and fat, see p.42

✗ deep-fried, see p.42

✓ thighs, boneless, skinless, uncooked, 170g (6oz), see p.42

✗ wings, see p.42

chocolate, see pp.128–9

✓ dark (minimum 70 per cent cocoa solids), 28g (1oz)

✗ milk

✗ white

coffee, see p.132 and Portion distortion, pp.134–5

✳ black, with sugar substitute, no milk, 237ml (8fl oz)

✗ cappuccino with full-fat milk and sugar

✗ with full-fat milk and sugar in large amounts

✗ frappe

✗ latte in large amounts

✳ with skimmed milk and 1 tsp sugar, 237ml (8fl oz)

cola, see pp.132–3

✳ diet, 237ml (8fl oz)

✗ regular

✓ coleslaw, 120g (4¼oz), see p.84

cookies, see p.127

✳ choc chip, 2, about 28g (1oz)

✓ wholegrain, 2, about 28g (1oz)

✳ cream, double, 1 tbsp, use only in balanced recipe, see p.62

✗ crisps, see p.141

croissant, see pp.105, 106

✳ plain, 28g (1oz)

✳ almond, 28g (1oz)

✗ chocolate

D

desserts, see pp.120–23

✳ apple pie, 57g (2oz)

✳ blackberry pie, 57g (2oz)

✳ bread pudding, 57g (2oz)

✳ carrot cake, 28g (1oz)

cheesecake

✳ chocolate, 28g (1oz)

✳ fruit, 28g (1oz)

✳ plain, 28g (1oz)

✳ chocolate cake, 28g (1oz)

✳ crème caramel, 57g (2oz)

✳ ice cream, see Ice cream

✳ peach cobbler, 57g (2oz)

✳ peach pie, 57g (2oz)

✳ pecan pie, 28g (1oz)

✳ pie, fruit, 57g (2oz)

✳ rhubarb pie, 57g (2oz)

✳ sorbet, fruit, 88g (3oz)

✳ tiramisu, 57g (2oz)

✳ drinks, diet 237ml (8fl oz), see pp.132–3

duck, see p.42

✳ with skin and visible fat removed, uncooked, 170g (6oz)

✗ with skin and fat

doughnut, see pp.106, 107

✳ plain, 28g (1oz)

✗ jam- or cream-filled

E

eggs, see pp.66–7

✓ 1–2

✗ fried in butter, bacon or sausage fat

F

fish

✓ cod, uncooked, 170g (6oz), see p.50

✗ deep-fried, see p.50

✓ flatfish (plaice or sole), uncooked, 170g (6oz), see p.50

✓ grey mullet, uncooked, 170g (6oz), see p.50

✓ grouper, uncooked, 170g (6oz), see p.50

✓ haddock, uncooked, 170g (6oz), see p.50

✓ hake, uncooked, 170g (6oz), see p.50

✓ halibut, uncooked, 170g (6oz), see p.50

✓ herring, uncooked, 170g (6oz), see p.52

✗ in batter, see p.50

✗ in breadcrumbs, see p.50

✓ john dory, uncooked, 170g (6oz), see p.50

✓ mackerel, uncooked, 170g (6oz), see p.52

✓ mahi-mahi, uncooked, 170g (6oz), see p.50

✓ monkfish, uncooked, 170g (6oz) see p.50

✓ orange roughy, uncooked, 170g (6oz), see p.50

✓ perch, uncooked, 170g (6oz), see p.50

✓ red mullet, uncooked, 170g (6oz), see p.50

✓ red snapper, uncooked, 170g (6oz), see p.50

✓ salmon, uncooked, 170g (6oz), see pp.52, 53

✓ sardines, uncooked, 170g (6oz), see p.52

✓ sea bass, uncooked, 170g (6oz), see p.50

✓ sea trout, uncooked, 170g (6oz), see p.50

✓ trout, uncooked, 170g (6oz), see p.52

✓ tuna, bluefin, yellowfin or albacore, uncooked, 170g (6oz), see pp.50, 52

✓ turbot, uncooked, 170g (6oz), see p.50

fruit, dried, see p.89

✳ apricots, 33g (1oz)

✽ figs, 37g (1¼oz)
✽ sultanas, 41g (1½oz)
fruit, fresh, per portion, *see* pp.86–9
  ✓ apples, 1 small
  ✓ apricots, 4 medium
  ✓ bananas, 1 x 20cm (8in)
  ✓ blackberries, 145g (5oz)
  ✓ blueberries, 145g (5oz)
  ✓ cherries, with stones, 117g (4oz)
  ✓ figs, 4
  ✓ grapefruit, 1 x 10cm (4in) diameter
  ✓ grapes, about 20
  ✓ kiwis, 2 small
  ✓ mangoes, 1 medium
  melon,
    ✓ cantaloupe, cubed, 160g (5¾oz)
    ✓ honeydew, cubed, 170g (6oz)
    ✓ watermelon, cubed, 152g (5½oz)
  ✓ nectarines, 1 medium
  ✓ oranges, 1 large
  ✓ papaya, cubed, 140g (5oz)
  ✓ peaches, 1 medium
  ✓ pears, 1 medium
  ✓ pineapple, cubed, 155g (5½oz)
  ✓ plums, 2 large
  ✓ raspberries, 123g (4½oz)
  ✓ strawberries, whole, 144g (5oz)
  ✓ tangerines, 2

G
✽ grape juice, unsweetened, 177ml (6fl oz), *see* pp.91, 132
✽ grapefruit juice, unsweetened, 177ml (6fl oz), *see* p.92

H, I
ham
  ✓ black forest, lean, 113g (4oz), lunch portion, *see* p.45
  ✓ lean, cured, 170g (6oz), *see* p.39
  ✗ regular (not lean), smoked or cured, *see* p.39

hamburgers, *see* Portion distortion, pp.36–7
✓ houmus, 2 tbsp, as snack, *see* pp.80, 81
ice cream, *see* Portion distortion, pp.124–5

J
✽ juice, fruit, unsweetened, 177ml (6fl oz), *see* pp.91, 132

L
lamb, *see* pp.40-41
  ✓ kebabs, cut from the leg or shoulder, uncooked, 170g (6oz)
  ✓ leg, uncooked, 170g (6oz)
    ✓ loin chops, uncooked, 170g (6oz)
    ✗ rib chops
    ✓ shoulder, uncooked, 170g (6oz)
legumes, cooked, 84–99g (3–3½oz)
depending on variety, *see* p.81
  ✓ black beans
  ✓ black-eyed beans
  ✓ butter beans
  ✓ cannellini beans
  ✓ chickpeas
  ✓ haricot beans
  ✓ kidney beans
  ✓ lentils
  ✓ pinto beans
  ✓ split peas

M
mayonnaise, *see* Dairy-based toppings p.62
milk, *see* p.58
  ✽ flavoured
  ✓ semi-skimmed, 237ml (8fl oz)
  ✓ skimmed, 237ml (8fl oz)
  ✗ whole
✗ mortadella, *see* p.45
✽ muffin, ½ mini, 28g (1oz), *see* p.104

N, O
✗ nachos, *see* p.65
nuts, *see* Vegetarian Options, p.47
oils, *see* p.85
  ✗ coconut
  ✓ olive, 1 tsp
  ✗ palm
  ✓ rapeseed, 1 tsp
  ✓ safflower, 1 tsp
  ✓ soya bean, 1 tsp
  ✓ sunflower, 1 tsp
✓ olives, 15, as snack, *see* p.141
✽ orange juice, unsweetened, 177ml (6fl oz), *see* pp.91, 132

P, Q
pasta, *see* pp.114–15
  ✗ cannelloni
  ✗ spaghetti carbonara
  ✗ fettuccine alfredo
  ✗ lasagne
  ✓ wholewheat, cooked, 170g (6oz), as side dish
✗ pastrami, *see* p.45
pastries, *see* pp.104–7
  croissant
    ✽ plain, 28g (1oz)
    ✽ almond, 28g (1oz)
    ✗ chocolate
  ✽ Danish pastry, 28g (1oz)
    ✗ with cheese
    ✗ with nuts
  ✽ doughnut 28g (1oz)
    ✗ jam-filled
    ✗ cream-filled
  ✽ muffin, ½ a mini, 28g (1oz)
    ✗ flapjacks
    ✗ sticky buns
peanuts
  ✓ butter, 2 tbsp, *see* p.101
  ✓ dry-roasted, as snack, 28g (1oz), *see* p.140
✓ pecans, as snack, 28g (1oz), *see* p.140
✽ pineapple juice, unsweetened, 177ml (6fl oz), *see* pp.91, 132

✓ pitta, wholemeal, 6in (15cm), *see* 195, 196

pizza, *see* Portion distortion, pp.116–17

popcorn, *see* Portion distortion, pp.142–3

pork
  ✗ bacon, *see* p.39
  ✳ bacon, back, uncooked, 170g (6oz), *see* p.39
  ✓ black forest ham, lean, 113g (4oz), lunch portion, *see* p.45
  ✓ ham, lean, cured, 170g (6oz), *see* p.39
  ✗ ham, regular, smoked or cured, *see* p.39
  ✓ loin chops, boneless, uncooked, 170g (6oz), *see* p.39
  ✳ loin roast, boneless, uncooked 170g (6oz), *see* p.39
  ✗ rinds, *see* p.39
  ✗ sausage, *see* p.39
  ✳ shoulder, uncooked, 170g (6oz), *see* p.39
  ✗ spareribs, *see* p.39
  ✓ tenderloin, uncooked, 170g (6oz), *see* p.39

poultry (*see* Chicken, Turkey, Duck)

✳ pretzels, 28g (1oz), as snack, *see* pp.140, 141

✳ prune juice, unsweetened, 177ml (6fl oz), *see* pp.91, 132

✓ quinoa, cooked, 157g (5³/₄oz), *see* pp.112–13

R

rice, *see* pp.112–13
  ✓ brown, cooked 146g (5¹/₄oz)
  ✗ fried, as a main dish
  ✗ risotto, as a main dish
  ✳ white, cooked, 119g (4¹/₄oz)
  ✓ wild, cooked, 123g (4¹/₂oz)

S

salad greens (eat freely), *see* p.82
✓ baby leaf spinach
✓ cos

✓ frisée
✓ iceberg
✓ lamb's lettuce
✓ little gem
✓ mizuna
✓ radicchio
✓ red leaf
✓ red mustard
✓ red oak leaf
✓ rocket
✓ romaine

salad dressings
  ✓ blue cheese, 1 tbsp, *see* p.85
  ✓ caesar, 1 tbsp, *see* p.85
  ✓ french, 1 tbsp, *see* p.83

salad extras, *see* p.82

salami, *see* p.45
  ✗ Genoa
  ✗ hard

seeds, *see* Vegetarian options p.47

✓ seitan, 57g (2oz), *see* p.47

shellfish, *see* pp.54–5
  ✗ au gratin
  ✓ clams, uncooked, 170g (6oz)
  ✓ crab, uncooked, 170g (6oz)
  ✓ crayfish, uncooked, 170g (6oz)
  ✗ deep-fried
  ✗ hollandaise
  ✗ in batter
  ✗ mornay
  ✓ lobster, uncooked, 170g (6oz)
  ✗ thermidor
  ✓ mussels, uncooked, 170g (6oz)
  ✓ octopus, uncooked, 170g (6oz)
  ✓ oysters, 170g (6oz)
  ✓ prawns, uncooked, 170g (6oz)
  ✓ scallops, uncooked, 170g (6oz)
  ✓ squid, uncooked, 170g (6oz)
  ✗ with breadcrumbs

✓ soya milk, fat-free or low-fat, 237ml (8fl oz), *see* p.58

spirits, *see* pp.136–7
  ✗ daiquiri, frozen
  ✓ gin, 44ml (1¹/₂fl oz)
  ✗ margarita
  ✗ mojito
  ✗ piña colada

✗ rum punch
✓ scotch, 44ml (1¹/₂fl oz)
✓ vodka, 44ml (1¹/₂fl oz)
✓ whisky, 44ml (1¹/₂fl oz)
  ✗ with tonic
✓ sweets, sugar-free or low-calorie, 28g (1oz), *see* p.128

T

tacos, *see* Portion distortion, pp.102–103

✓ tahini, 2 tbsp, *see* p.47

tea, *see* p.132
  ✓ black, unsweetened
  ✳ black, with 1 tsp sugar and skimmed milk, 237ml (8fl oz)
  ✳ chai, 237ml (8fl oz)
  ✓ green, unsweetened
  ✓ herbal, unsweetened
  ✳ ice, instant, with 1 tsp sugar, 237ml (8fl oz)
  ✓ red, unsweetened

✓ tempeh, 113g (4oz), *see* p.47

✓ textured vegetable protein (TVP), 57g (2oz), *see* p.47

tofu, *see* p.47
  ✗ deep-fried
  ✓ firm, 170g (6oz)
  ✓ soft, 170g (6oz)

✓ tomato juice, low-salt, 237ml (8fl oz), *see* p.70

✳ tortilla chips, as snack, 28g (1oz), *see* p.141

✓ tortilla, flour, 15cm (6in), *see* p.96

turkey
  ✓ breast, boneless, skinless, uncooked, 170g (6oz), *see* p.42
  ✗ breast with skin and fat, *see* p.42
  ✓ breast, skinless, lower-sodium slices, cooked, 113g (4oz), lunch portion, *see* p.45
  ✗ dark meat with skin and fat, *see* p.42
  ✓ thighs, boneless, skinless, uncooked, 170g (6oz), *see* p.42

V

vegetable juice, low salt, 237ml (8fl oz), *see* p.70
vegetables (you can eat freely of those marked ✓)
- ✓ artichokes, *see* p.71
- ✓ asparagus, *see* p.71
- ✓ aubergine, *see* p.71
- ✓ bean sprouts, *see* p.71
- ✓ bok choy, *see* p.71
- ✓ broccoli, *see* pp.70, 71
- ✓ brussels sprouts, *see* p.71
- ✓ cabbage, red, *see* p.71
- ✓ cabbage, white, *see* p.71
- ✓ carrots, *see* p.71
- ✓ cauliflower, *see* p.71
- ✓ celery, *see* p.71
- ✓ chinese cabbage, *see* p.71
- ✓ courgettes, *see* p.71
- ✓ cucumber, *see* p.71
- ✓ garlic, *see* p.71
- ✓ green beans, *see* p.71
- ✓ kale, *see* p.71
- ✓ kohl rabi, *see* p.71
- ✓ lettuce (all types), *see* pp.71, 82
- ✓ mushrooms, *see* p.71
- ✓ okra, *see* p.71
- ✓onions, *see* p.71
- ✲ parsnips, uncooked, 67g (2½oz), *see* p.72
- ✲ peas, uncooked, 73g (2¾oz), see pp.72, 73
- ✓ peppers, green, red and yellow, *see* p.71
- potatoes
  - ✲ baked, 113–170g (4–6oz), *see* p.75, and Portion distortion pp.78–9
  - ✲ boiled, 113–170g (4–6oz), *see* p.75
  - ✲ chips, *see* Portion distortion, pp.74–5
  - ✲ crisps, as snack, 28g (1oz), *see* p.141
  - ✲ mashed, 113–170g (4–6oz), *see* pp.75
  - ✲ salad, 125g (4½ oz), *see* p.84
  - ✲ sauté, 113–170g (4–6oz), *see* pp.75
  - ✲ steamed, 113–170g (4–6oz), *see* pp.75
  - ✲ sweet, uncooked, 67g (2½oz), *see* p.72
- ✓ pumpkin, *see* p.71
- ✓ radishes, *see* p.71
- ✓ runner beans, *see* p.71
- ✓ spinach, *see* p.71
- ✓ spring greens, *see* p.71
- squash
  - ✓ acorn
  - ✓ butternut
  - ✓ spaghetti
  - ✓ yellow
- ✲ sweetcorn, uncooked, 72g (2¾oz), *see* pp.72, 73
- ✓ tomatoes, *see* p.71
- ✲ yam, uncooked, 73g (2¾oz)

✓ vegetable juice, low-salt, 237ml (8fl oz), *see* p.71

W

✓ walnuts, as snack, 28g (1oz), *see* p.140
wine, *see* p.137 and Portion distortion, pp.138–9
- ✓ red, 148ml (5fl oz)
- ✓ white, 148ml (5fl oz)

Y

yogurt, *see* pp.58–9 and Portion distortion, pp.60–1
- ✲ frozen, sugar-free, fat-free, 72g (2¾oz)
- ✗ full-fat
- ✗ fruit-flavoured, sweetened
- ✗ granola-topped
- ✓ fat-free, low-sugar, 227g (8oz)
- ✓ fat-free, fruit-flavoured, 227g (8oz)
- ✗ drink, sweetened
- ✗ whole milk

Web-based resources

Interested in learning more about the food we eat and how what we eat affects our health? Below are some helpful food and health-related websites from the UK, Australia, the USA, and Canada.

UNITED KINGDOM

www.food.gov.uk
The Food Standards Agency (FSA) provides advice and information to the public and government on food safety, nutrition and diet. It also protects consumers through effective food enforcement and monitoring.

www.eatwell.gov.uk
Much of the FSA's advice on diet and health is on their Eatwell website. It offers reliable and practical advice about healthy eating, understanding food labels and how what we eat can affect our health.

www.cancerindex.org
Cancer-UK is an independent non-profit website which aims to provide both an overview and a gateway to UK-based cancer resources such as Cancer Research UK, Macmillan Cancer Support, CancerBackup and Marie Curie Cancer Care.

www.diabetes.org.uk/home.htm
Diabetes UK is the largest organization in the UK working for people with diabetes, funding research, campaigning and helping people live with the condition. Their website provides detailed and factual information on all aspects of living with diabetes.

www.bhf.org.uk
The British Heart Foundation (BHF) is the largest independent funder of heart research in the UK. Its website offers information on heart conditions, healthy eating, cholesterol and other heart-health issues, and offers a heart information helpline.

www.healthyliving.gov.uk
This joint collaboration between Health Scotland and the Scottish Executive promotes Scotland's healthy living programme, but is suitable for anyone who wishes to achieve a healthier diet and a more active lifestyle. It provides resources, advice and support on healthy eating and physical activity.

www.patient.co.uk
This website aims to provide non-medical people in the UK with good-quality information about health and disease. It offers downloadable information leaflets on a wide range of medical and health topics.

AUSTRALIA

www.foodstandards.gov.au
Food Standards Australia New Zealand (FSANZ) develops effective food standards. Visit this site to learn the latest about what's in the food you eat, how to interpret health claims and how to read food labels.

www.healthinsite.gov.au
HealthInsite is an initiative of the Australian government. It provides up-to-date information on health topics as well as the latest recommendations for fitness and nutrition through links to authoritative websites and articles.

www.nutritionaustralia.org
A non-government, non-profit, community-based organization that provides scientific nutrition information to encourage all Australians to achieve optimal health through food variety and physical activity. Use this site to find out the latest information on nutrition for all ages and facts about food.

www.health.gov.au
Visit the Australian Government Department for Health and Ageing site for information and help about medical conditions and diseases, health products and medicines, healthcare systems, ageing, rural health services, ethical issues and gene technology.

www.heartfoundation.com.au
The Heart Foundation website provides news and information on recent research, advice on healthy lifestyles and facts about heart diseases and conditions, as well as

guidelines and other resources for health professionals. It also offers fun ways to promote heart health.

www.diabetesaustralia.com.au
The Diabetes Australia site provides information on research, news and events, offers diabetes guidelines and a range of fact sheets, as well as links to relevant organizations.

www.cancer.org.au
The Cancer Council Australia is the country's national non-government cancer control organization. It promotes cancer research and provides information and support for people affected by cancer. Go to this site to find out about prevention and early detection, patient support and the latest treatments.

USA
www.MyPyramid.gov
Go to this site to help you choose the foods and amounts that are right for you. The United States Department of Agriculture (USDA) released the MyPyramid food guidance system to educate consumers and to help them make the right food choices.

www.5aday.gov
The 5 A Day for Better Health Programme is a national initiative to increase public awareness of the importance of eating a minimum of five, and preferably nine servings, of fruits and vegetables a day. It gives tips on how to include more fruits and vegetables in your daily diet.

www.nal.usda.gov/fnic/foodcomp/search/
Use the USDA National Nutrient Database to find the nutritional value of foods. It is the foundation of most food and nutrition databases in the US and is used in food policy, research and nutrition.

www.cfsan.fda.gov/~dms/foodlab.html
This website is useful if you are confused about nutritional labels. It gives tips on how to effectively and easily read nutritional labels.

www.foodsafety.gov
This site gives up-to-date US government food safety advice on what's safe and what isn't in our food supply.

www.cancer.org
The American Cancer Society is a nationwide, community-based voluntary health organization. It gives information about preventing and fighting cancer.

www.diabetes.org
This site for The American Diabetes Association provides information about diabetes. The association conducts programmes throughout the US geared to preventing and curing diabetes and to improving the lives of all people affected by diabetes.

www.americanheart.org
This is the site for The American Heart Association. It gives information on how to prevent and manage cardiovascular diseases and stroke.

CANADA
www.hc-sc.gc.ca
The Health Canada website links to Canada's Food Guide to Healthy Living, which provides information on food safety, labelling and nutrition.

www.healthyeatingisinstore.ca
The Canadian Diabetes Association and Dieticians of Canada have teamed up to bring consumers a user-friendly website to better understand nutrition labelling and make healthy food choices.

www.inspection.gc.ca
The Canadian Food Inspection Agency (CFIA) is Canada's federal food safety, animal health and plant protection agency. Their website provides fact sheets and reference materials on labelling practices, food safety, consumer protection and food allergens.

www.cancer.ca
The Canadian Cancer Society provides information on cancer prevention and early detection. It also provides services and support to patients and family members.

www.diabetes.ca
The Canadian Diabetes Association is dedicated to improving the lives of people with diabetes through education, research and clinical care. Their website offers nutrition guides, meal plans and tips for healthy eating, as well as information on diabetes prevention and management.

www.heartandstroke.ca
The Canadian Heart and Stroke Foundation's website offers consumers information on healthy living, including making heart-smart food choices.

Index

Acknowledgments

Author's acknowledgments Many thanks and much love go to my husband, Harold. His guidance and advice on every page helped me to complete this project. His constant support for all of my work has been a delight for me.

Lisa Ekus as my friend and agent encouraged and helped me to bring this book to publication. Lisa, thank you and great working with you.

This book would not have come about without the insight of Mary-Clare Jerram whose timely visit to the US brought us together and brought life to the concept.

Thanks also to Carl Raymond for his active participation and enthusiasm for the project.

Thanks to the staff at DK and editors Jenny Latham and Hilary Mandleberg.

I'd also like to thank my family who have always supported my projects and encouraged me every step of the way: My son James, his wife Patty, and their children, Zachary, Jacob and Haley who gave advice; my son John, his wife Jill and their children Jeffrey and Joanna who cheered me on; my son Charles, his wife Lori and their sons, Daniel and Matthew for their guidance. my sister Roberta and brother-in-law Robert who provide a continuous sounding board for my ideas.

I'd like to thank the many readers who correspond with me to say how much they enjoy my work. This kind of encouragement makes the solitary time in front of the computer worthwhile. You can continue to contact me through my website **www.DinnerInMinutes.com.**

Publisher's acknowledgments Dorling Kindersley would like to thank photographer Sian Irvine and her assistant Byll Pullman; home economist Sarah Tildesley and her assistant Claire Ptak; Ruth Hope for the styling; Sue Bosanko for the index; Kathy Steer for additional editorial assistance and proof-reading; Vicky Read for design assistance; Sonia Charbonnier for all her DTP support.

Symbols artwork by Joanna Cameron

Picture credits

Linda Gassenheimer is a TV and radio personality, syndicated journalist, best-selling author of over twelve books, spokesperson and food consultant. Her *Low-Carb Meals in Minutes* reached number one on Amazon.com's best-seller list for all books and number two on the LA Times Hot Books list. It has been published in the UK, where it reached number one on the www.amazon.co.uk best-seller list, and in Norway, New Zealand and Australia.

Linda is the producer and host of the weekly feature, Food News and Views, on WLRN 91.3FM National Public Radio for South Florida, and has made guest appearances on numerous radio and television programmes throughout the United States and Canada. These include Television Food Network, most recently with Sarah Moulton on Cooking Live and Sara's Secrets, Good Morning America, Cookin' USA, The Low Cholesterol Gourmet, Canada AM, and she had her own feature called Dinner in Minutes on the Miami NBC TV affiliate.

Her column on www.Miami Herald.com, 'Dinner in Minutes', is read by over four million readers. In addition, she writes regularly for Bottom Line Newspaper and has written for *Prevention Magazine*, *Food and Wine*, *Cooking Light*, *LowCarb Living* and several other national publications.

Linda's credentials include an advanced Cordon Bleu degree, training with a two-star chef in France for three years, cooking training with Simone Beck in the South of France and with Marcella Hazan at her cooking school in Bologna, Italy, and ten years' experience as Executive Director of a chain of gourmet supermarkets in Miami. She developed and ran CuisinEase cooking school in London for nine years.